C000081269

YOUR
ARTERIES

AN OWNER'S MANUAL

WILLIAM L. DRISCOLL

Based on 40 groundbreaking
medical journal articles

Hawkeye Press
Virginia

This book, based on 40 medical journal articles, is meant to inform everyone with arteries. It is not intended as medical advice and does not take the place of medical advice or treatment from a doctor. Readers should consult their health care provider for specific health concerns and questions. This book is not a diagnostic tool and cannot be used to suggest, confirm, contradict or rule out any medical diagnosis. While the author has done his best to ensure that the information presented here is up to date as of the time of publication, research is ongoing and it is possible that new findings may either challenge or reinforce some of the information presented here.

CONTENTS

1

HEART DISEASE IS A DISEASE
OF THE ARTERIES

The disease known as heart disease is better understood as a disease of the arteries.

To have the best chance of preventing heart disease, it's helpful to understand how changes in the arteries over time can result in a heart attack, a stroke, or other health problems.

A heart attack happens when an artery serving the heart becomes blocked, preventing sufficient oxygen-rich blood from reaching the heart muscle.

A stroke happens when an artery to the brain becomes blocked, preventing sufficient blood from reaching the brain.

Heart disease is the leading cause of death both in the United States and worldwide.

Heart attacks and strokes are so common largely because the health of the arteries declines without causing symptoms until the problem has reached an advanced stage. Many people don't know they have heart disease until they have a heart attack or stroke. Tragically, sometimes a patient dies from their first heart attack or stroke.

The good news is that declining artery health can be detected at an early stage and treated before it causes a heart attack, stroke, or other health problems. For those found to have an early stage of heart disease, treatment with a statin medication or sometimes a newer medicine is very effective.

Current medical practice is to offer a statin prescription only after a patient's 10-year predicted risk from heart disease exceeds a certain level. Yet researchers found that a commonly used method to predict risk failed to prompt statin therapy in 85% of people in whom heart disease had already begun. Their study was published in the *Journal of the American College of Cardiology* in 2020.

Two heart doctors later said that relying on a method to predict risk allows heart disease "to proceed unchecked for decades," in an editorial published by the *Journal of the American Medical Association* in 2022.

Fortunately, early detection of heart disease is available with a noninvasive ultrasound test of the arteries in the neck. It's like the ultrasound test that pregnant women get, but on the neck instead of the belly.

Although few doctors and other primary care providers routinely offer patients this ultrasound screening, anyone can seek out the screening, as described in this book. For those who have early-stage heart disease, early detection makes early treatment possible.

Arteries to the Heart and Brain

Heart disease begins with artery clogging, a gradual process that continues for decades unless it is stopped through statin therapy, healthy lifestyle choices, or both.

The image on the next page from the U.S. National Institutes of Health compares a healthy artery to one that has become badly clogged with plaque.

The NIH explains that if an area of plaque bursts, "a blood clot may form that may block the artery completely or travel to other parts of the body. Blockages, either complete or incomplete, can cause complications, including heart attack, stroke, [and] vascular dementia."

A stroke, sometimes called a brain attack, is similar to a heart attack and causes part of the brain to die.

Vascular dementia, characterized by a decline in brain function and with symptoms like Alzheimer's disease, is caused by mini-strokes over time.

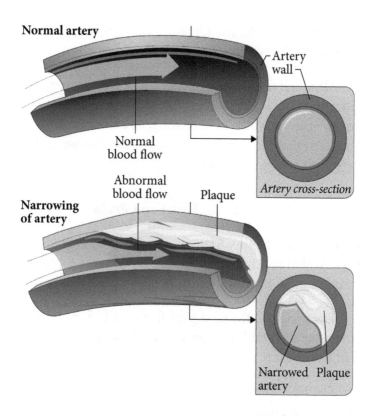

Normal artery

Artery wall

Normal blood flow

Artery cross-section

Abnormal blood flow

Plaque

Narrowing of artery

Narrowed artery   Plaque

Heart disease is also known as "cardiovascular" disease—which is a short way of saying "heart and blood vessel disease," because "cardio" means heart and "vascular" refers to blood vessels, such as arteries.

One type of heart disease, known as coronary artery disease, is caused by a buildup of plaque in the two coronary arteries, which supply oxygen-rich blood to the heart muscle.

A coronary artery is shown in the center of the following image from the U.S. Centers for Disease Control. If one of the coronary arteries becomes partly or completely blocked due to a plaque rupture, a heart attack can result.

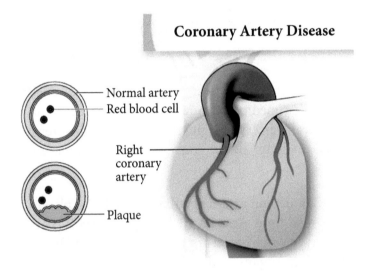

Coronary Artery Disease

Two other arteries, called carotid arteries, supply oxygen-rich blood to the brain. If one of these arteries gets clogged, a stroke can result.

A carotid artery is shown in the following image from the U.S. National Institutes of Health. The image highlights the point at which the carotid artery separates into two smaller arteries.

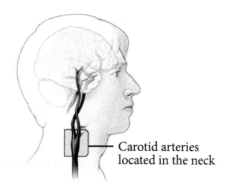

Carotid arteries
located in the neck

Another name for heart disease or cardiovascular disease is the medical term "atherosclerosis," which literally means artery clogging. The plain English term "artery clogging" better conveys what this disease is about.

It's about your arteries getting clogged with plaque, slowly, over time. Arteries are hugely important. They carry oxygen-rich blood not just to the heart and brain, but to all the organs, and every part of the body.

Beyond heart attacks, strokes and vascular dementia, artery clogging can cause other health problems as well.

Artery clogging can lead to kidney disease, peripheral artery disease, impaired sexual response, and "poor aging due to loss of function in multiple organs," according to a state-of-the-art review article by Professor Michael Makover at NYU Grossman

School of Medicine and two co-authors, published in the *American Journal of Preventive Cardiology*.

The Changing View of Artery Clogging

Artery clogging was seen in the past as "an inevitable, degenerative accompaniment to aging," wrote cardiologist (heart specialist) Peter Libby, a Harvard Medical School professor, in an article published in the scientific journal *Nature* in 2021.

But now we know, he said, that lifestyle and medical measures can "modulate" the disease process, and that the disease can even "regress." He said that LDL cholesterol "causes atherosclerosis," or artery clogging. LDL is known as the "bad" type of cholesterol.

Researchers have found that artery clogging is common in healthy adults as young as their mid-40s, as discussed in chapter 2. For some individuals, artery clogging may start at an earlier age.

Benefits of Screening for Artery Clogging

Five cardiologists have recommended artery screening to detect early-stage artery clogging, in an article published in the *Journal of the American College of Cardiology* in 2019, as discussed in chapter 4.

If plaque in the arteries is found, intensive statin therapy can reduce the level of LDL cholesterol in the blood to a level low enough to "halt" plaque progression, the cardiologists said, and thereby reduce the likelihood of a heart attack or stroke.

The U.S. Preventive Services Task Force has made a compelling argument for screening the carotid arteries in the neck, saying that plaque in the carotid arteries "is a manifestation of systemic disease, so identifying this condition may potentially lead to changes in medical management to prevent future cardiovascular events," such as heart attacks and strokes.

The task force report that made that argument is discussed in chapter 4.

Ultrasound Artery Screening

A carotid artery ultrasound screening test is one means to detect artery clogging at the earliest stage. The screening test is widely available without a doctor's order, as discussed in chapter 5. Unlike a medical X-ray or CT scan, an ultrasound test does not involve ionizing radiation and is therefore very safe. Another type of screening test, known as a coronary artery calcium (CAC) scan, requires a doctor's order and is not considered in this book.

If Screening Identifies Artery Clogging

If you obtain a carotid artery ultrasound screening test and it shows that your arteries are getting clogged, you can talk to your primary care provider about two steps that can slow or stop the progression of artery clogging or even reverse it somewhat. Those two steps are healthy lifestyle changes, and a prescription for a statin drug.

Healthier habits, a statin medication, or both work to prevent artery clogging by reducing the level of "bad" LDL cholesterol in the blood.

LDL cholesterol in the blood has been found to cause artery clogging, and is seen as the strongest modifiable risk factor for the disease, as described in chapter 2.

Healthy lifestyle changes are described in chapter 6. These changes, although they can be difficult to make, can be quite effective.

There may be some individuals for whom a healthier diet or other lifestyle changes may be sufficient to reduce the level of LDL in the blood low enough to reach their goal—for example, to reach an LDL level low enough to stop the progression of artery clogging.

Yet for many people, lifestyle changes may not be possible or may not sufficiently protect the arteries. That's where statins can help. Statin therapy can reduce the level of LDL cholesterol in the blood by as much as 50% or possibly more, as discussed in chapter 7.

Moreover, statins can stabilize existing plaque in the arteries, which can help prevent a heart attack or stroke.

Cardiologists in the U.S. and Europe agree that statins are generally safe, as described in chapter 8.

Purpose of This Book

This book is designed to be an owner's manual for your arteries.

Especially from middle age onward, our arteries may require preventive maintenance. While there's no on-board diagnostic system for our arteries, as there is for motor vehicles, a widely available screening test can show when preventive maintenance is needed.

This book begins with chapters on how arteries get clogged, why that's bad for your health, whether to get screened for artery clogging, and how to do so.

For those who discover from a screening test that their arteries are getting clogged, this book discusses options to prevent a heart attack by stabilizing existing artery-clogging plaque and slowing, stopping, or even reversing the progression of artery clogging.

A chapter on healthy lifestyle choices describes what can be done without medication. Two chapters on statin therapy, which a doctor or other primary care provider may prescribe, discuss statin effectiveness and safety.

A final chapter describes the role of preventive cardiologists, who can prescribe a level of statin medication that could prevent further artery clogging. Help in finding a preventive cardiologist is provided in the appendix.

This book is based on research published in 40 groundbreaking medical journal articles. Each article was written by a team of doctors and reviewed by other doctors before being published in a medical journal.

A "notes" section at the end of the book provides details on the medical research discussed. Many of the most significant journal articles are available online for free.

Highlights Ahead

Here are some highlights from the chapters ahead:

Chapter 2: For "bad" LDL cholesterol, the lower the longer, the better.

Chapter 3: Artery clogging can slow down your brain.

Chapter 4: Five cardiologists (heart specialists) have proposed testing people for artery clogging. Also, the Mayo Clinic and Cleveland Clinic suggest a carotid artery ultrasound examination for those with high blood pressure.

Chapter 5: Ultrasound screening for artery clogging is available without a doctor's order.

Chapter 6: The American Heart Association recommends eight healthy habits that can protect the health of your arteries.

Chapter 7: Statin therapy can prevent a heart attack by stabilizing existing artery-clogging plaque. It can also slow, stop, or potentially reverse artery clogging.

Chapter 8: American and European cardiologists agree that statins are generally safe.

Chapter 9: A preventive cardiologist can prescribe a level of statin medication that could help you achieve a longer, healthier life.

Appendix: Preventive cardiologists work at dozens of health care systems around the U.S.

2

HOW ARTERIES GET CLOGGED
EVEN WITH A "NORMAL"
CHOLESTEROL LEVEL

The form of cholesterol known as "bad" LDL cholesterol causes artery clogging, which leads to heart disease.

The European Atherosclerosis Society Consensus Panel presented that conclusion using medical language, saying that LDL particles in the blood "cause atherosclerotic cardiovascular disease," in a statement published in the *European Heart Journal* in 2017.

Building on that understanding, researchers found that a high level of LDL cholesterol was the "strongest modifiable risk factor" for artery clogging, in a study published in the *Journal of the American College of Cardiology* in 2020. (For details on all studies, see the "notes" section at the end of this book.)

The level of LDL in the blood is determined by a blood test called a cholesterol panel or "lipid panel," which your primary care provider can order and which testing labs such as Quest and LabCorp may offer in your area without a doctor's order.

Whether or not you know your current level of LDL cholesterol, it is worth understanding what medical researchers have discovered about how various levels of LDL can affect your health.

For many people, even an average level of LDL in the blood results in artery clogging. People with an above-average level of LDL or other risk factors are at higher risk for artery clogging.

But if you find out that your arteries are getting clogged, you can take action to reduce your LDL cholesterol level.

LDL cholesterol can be reduced in two ways, potentially adding healthy years to your life: by taking on additional healthy lifestyle choices, if possible (see chapter 6), and through treatment with a statin medication, which can lower LDL by as much as 50% or possibly more (see chapter 7).

Research has shown that reducing your LDL to a relatively low level could slow or stop artery clogging, or even reverse it somewhat (see chapter 7).

If an ultrasound artery screening test shows that you have artery clogging, knowing the health effects of various levels of LDL can be helpful in a discussion with your doctor about an appropriate target level for your LDL to limit or prevent further artery clogging.

This chapter is intended to help you gain an understanding of the health effects of various levels of LDL cholesterol in the blood, by presenting the findings of medical research. Because some of these research findings are recent, your primary care provider may not be fully aware of them.

For "Bad" LDL Cholesterol, "Lower is Better"

Five cardiologists and other researchers published an influential article nearly 20 years ago concluding that an LDL level below 70 mg/dL (milligrams per deciliter) is best.

(If you live outside the U.S. and your LDL level is measured in different units, you may consult the conversion table at the end of this chapter.)

The five researchers compiled data showing that LDL cholesterol ranges from 50 to 70 mg/dL for native hunter-gatherers, healthy human newborn children, primates in their natural habitat, and other wild mammals, "all of whom do not develop atherosclerosis."

Data from clinical trials through 2004, the authors wrote, "suggest" that the progression of artery clogging and the likelihood of heart attacks are minimized when LDL is lowered to less than 70 mg/dL.

The article advises that when it comes to LDL, "lower is better." Since the article was published in the *Journal of the American College of Cardiology* in 2004, it has been cited by more than 600 other journal articles.

Three cardiologists and other researchers raised the topic again in 2012, posing the question: When helping patients reduce their LDL level, "how low should we go?" Based on a review of the medical literature, they gave their answer in the title of their article: "LDL cholesterol: the lower the better."

The authors concluded that the "critical role" of lowering LDL cholesterol in reducing cardiovascular risk "is firmly established." Lowering the LDL level reduces the likelihood of heart attacks and strokes, they said, while slowing and "even inducing regression" of artery clogging. The article was published in the journal *Medical Clinics of North America* in 2012.

For "Bad" LDL Cholesterol, the Lower the *Longer*, the Better

A lower LDL level beginning early in life results in a "3-fold greater reduction" in the risk of coronary artery disease than lowering LDL to the same level beginning later in life, according to a study by 10 researchers published in the *Journal of the American College of Cardiology* in 2012.

The researchers reviewed health outcomes for those with genetic variations giving them low lifetime LDL levels, compared to those treated later in life with a statin medication to reduce their LDL level.

Commenting on the research findings, Peter Toth, director of preventive cardiology at CGH Medical Center in Illinois, said that the risk reduction from lowering LDL cholesterol is "proportional to both the magnitude of the reduction and the duration of time over which this reduction is sustained," in an article published in the *American Journal of Preventive Cardiology* in 2020.

"The reticence for treating patients, including young patients, with statins needs to end," he said.

Three researchers agreed two years later, concluding that "the earlier elevated LDL cholesterol is lowered, the better," in a state-of-the-art review article published in the *American Journal of Preventive Cardiology* in 2022.

People with LDL Levels as Low as 14 Experience a Significant Reduction in "Cardiovascular Events"

Eight doctors have reported that people with a genetic variation giving them "very low" LDL levels—as low as 14 mg/dL—have a "lifelong reduction" in their LDL level, are healthy, do not have any apparent illnesses related to their low LDL level, and "experience a significant reduction in cardiovascular events over long-term follow-up." (The genetic variation that results in these very low LDL levels is known as PCSK9 loss-of-function variation.)

The article, based on a review of previous medical research, was published in the *European Heart Journal* in 2021.

Some Preventive Cardiologists Aim for an LDL Level Below 38 in Patients with Artery Clogging

Some preventive cardiologists aim for much lower levels of LDL in patients with artery clogging than the level "below 100" that is still described by some in the medical community as "optimal," according to a standard that dates back to 2008.

Professor Michael Makover at the NYU Grossman School of Medicine and two co-authors said that "the goal" for LDL when plaque is present in the arteries should be below 38 mg/dL. Those with "major plaque," prior cardiovascular events, or other factors "will in most cases require lowering LDL cholesterol to below 20 mg/dL," the authors said. Their state-of-the-art review article was published in the *American Journal of Preventive Cardiology* in 2022.

At LDL Levels Above 40, the Risk of Coronary Artery Disease Increases at an Ever-Steeper Rate

In a highly influential study, nine researchers teamed with the Coordinating Committee of the National Cholesterol Education Program, managed by the U.S. National Institutes of Health, on a study that found that the risk of coronary artery disease rises with increasing LDL levels, and that the rate of increase in risk "rises more steeply" at higher LDL levels.

Their review article reached that finding by analyzing five "major clinical trials" of statin therapy whose results were published between 2001 and 2004.

The researchers said that starting from an LDL level of 40 mg/dL, for every 30 mg/dL increase above that level, "the data suggest" that the relative risk for coronary artery disease increases in proportion by about 30%.

The article, published in the *Journal of the American College of Cardiology* in 2004, has since been cited by 9,700 other studies.

European Guidelines from 2019 Recommend an LDL Level Below 55 in Patients with "Very High" Risk

The European Society of Cardiology and the European Atherosclerosis Society recommended in their

2019 cholesterol guidelines that for those at "very high" cardiovascular risk, the baseline LDL level should be reduced by at least 50%, and if the resulting LDL level is 55 mg/dL or above, the LDL level should be further reduced to achieve a level below 55 mg/dL.

The guidelines consider persons with "very high" risk to "generally" include those with documented heart disease due to artery clogging, type 1 or type 2 diabetes mellitus, very high levels of individual risk factors, or chronic kidney disease.

"Optimal LDL is 50 to 70"
According to a 2004 Study

An influential article described earlier in this chapter compiled evidence on the optimal LDL level, and stated its conclusion in the article's title: "Optimal low-density lipoprotein is 50 to 70 mg/dL: lower is better and physiologically normal."

The authors of that article said artery clogging is widespread in the U.S. "because the average person's LDL level is approximately twice the normal physiological level."

Existing Artery-Clogging Plaque
Can Regress at LDL Levels Below 70

A study by 26 researchers found that artery-clogging plaque regressed in study participants whose LDL level was reduced to 70 mg/dL or below. Artery blockage due to plaque, measured as a percentage of the artery's cross-section, regressed by up to two percentage points within the first year.

The study presented original research comparing the effects of a statin to the effects of a statin plus the drug ezetimibe, which also lowers LDL cholesterol, and described three previous studies on the effects of a statin alone.

Across the four studies, when the LDL cholesterol level was reduced to 70 mg/dL or below, the percentage of artery blockage was reduced on average across all participants during the time period of each study.

The authors also cited four research trials that showed that "mean LDL cholesterol levels were closely correlated with median change" in plaque volume.

Regarding the effects of prescribing two medicines at once, the authors found that median LDL levels after treatment with a statin plus ezetimibe were about 8 to 15 points lower than after treatment with a statin alone.

The study was published in the *Journal of the American College of Cardiology* in 2015.

American Guideline Recommends an LDL Level Below 70 for Most Patients with Heart Disease

Eleven doctors and researchers, including the lead author of the 2018 cholesterol management guideline from the American Heart Association and the American College of Cardiology, have noted that the guideline calls for patients with heart disease due to artery clogging to reduce their LDL level by 50% or more.

Most of those patients will have a baseline LDL level of less than 140, they wrote, so if they achieved the recommended "50% or more" reduction, the resulting LDL level for most patients would be less than 70 mg/dL (because half of 140 is 70).

The article was published in the journal *Mayo Clinic Proceedings* in 2021.

Among Healthy People with an LDL Level of 70-80, Nearly One-Fifth Had Artery Clogging by Their Mid-40s

Eleven researchers found in a study of middle-aged people without risk factors for cardiovascular disease that among those with an LDL level of 70-80 mg/dL, nearly one in five had artery clogging by their mid-40s.

The study was published in the *Journal of the American College of Cardiology* in 2017.

(The study is further described later in this chapter in a section discussing its main finding that most healthy people with an LDL level between 130 and 160 mg/dL had artery clogging by their mid-40s.)

An LDL Level Below 100 is Not
Protective Against Cardiovascular Disease

Eight researchers analyzed data on 136,000 patients hospitalized with coronary artery disease and concluded that an LDL level below 100 mg/dL is not protective against cardiovascular disease. Their study was published in the *American Heart Journal* in 2009.

"Almost half" of those patients had an LDL level at the time of hospital admission below 100 mg/dL, the co-authors found.

Coronary artery disease, also called coronary heart disease, is caused by a buildup of plaque in the two coronary arteries that deliver oxygen-rich blood to the heart muscle, as described in chapter 1.

An LDL Level of 115-120 Results
in 3x Higher Risk for "Adverse Outcomes"
than an LDL Level of 80-90

Three researchers found that the likelihood of "advanced cardiovascular disease" or death was 2.97 times higher among people with an LDL level of 115-120 mg/dL, than among people with an LDL level of 80-90 mg/dL, in a study published in the *Journal of the American Heart Association* in 2019.

The study examined the likelihood of "advanced cardiovascular disease" and the likelihood of death from all causes, among 3,875 participants, using data collected over an eight-year period.

Among Healthy People with an LDL Level of 130 to 160, Most Had Artery Clogging by Their Mid-40s

A study of middle-aged people without risk factors for cardiovascular disease found that among those with a moderately high level of LDL—between 130 and 160 mg/dL—most had artery clogging by their mid-40s.

The 1,779 men and women in the study, nearly all in their 40s, each had an LDL level lower than 160 and had none of four major risk factors for cardiovascular disease: high blood pressure, diabetes, a history of smoking, or a family history of cardiovascular disease.

The results of the study, as shown in the bar chart below, demonstrate that the likelihood of artery clogging increases at higher levels of LDL cholesterol in the blood.

Percentage of subjects, most in their 40s, with artery clogging at increasing LDL levels

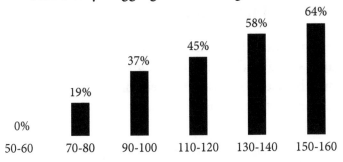

LDL cholesterol level (intermediate data not shown)

Across all 1,779 individuals studied, 30% had plaque in the arteries supplying blood to the legs, 23% had plaque in the carotid arteries supplying blood to the brain, 17% had plaque in the abdominal aorta (the final section of the aorta, the body's largest artery), and 11% had calcified plaque in the coronary arteries that supply oxygenated blood to the heart.

Researchers tested the first three artery locations using ultrasound, and tested the coronary arteries using a coronary artery calcium test. They found that 23% had plaque in just one location, 21% had plaque in two or three locations, and 6% had plaque in four or more locations.

While this study evaluated subjects with no major risk factors, the researchers also noted a previous study they had conducted of a group of middle-aged men and women at "low" risk of cardiovascular disease, which found that nearly 60% had arterial plaque in at least one location, and 41% had plaque in two or more locations.

An editorial comment published along with the study suggests that arterial imaging at an early stage could be used to guide treatment decisions that could help prevent cardiovascular disease.

An LDL Level of 160 to 189 Represents Another Step Higher in Risk

A study discussed early in this chapter found that for every 30 mg/dL increase in the LDL level, the risk for coronary artery disease increases by about 30% beyond the risk level for those with an LDL level 30 points lower.

At an LDL Level of 190 or Higher, Medical Guidelines Recommend High-Intensity Statin Therapy

For patients with an LDL level of 190 mg/dL or higher, the American College of Cardiology and American Heart Association recommend beginning "high-intensity" statin therapy on that basis alone, in clinical practice guidelines set in 2018.

The dosage of any statin medication is classified as "high intensity" if it reduces the LDL level by at least 50% on average (see chapter 7).

Table to Convert an LDL Level Measured in mg/dL to an LDL Level Measured in mmol/L

For those who live in a region where LDL cholesterol is measured in units of mmol/L, the following table may be helpful.

LDL cholesterol in mg/dL		LDL cholesterol in mmol/L
40 mg/dL	equals	1.0 mmol/L
70 mg/dL	equals	1.8 mmol/L
100 mg/dL	equals	2.6 mmol/L
130 mg/dL	equals	3.4 mmol/L
160 mg/dL	equals	4.1 mmol/L
190 mg/dL	equals	4.9 mmol/L

3

LIMITING ARTERY CLOGGING AT AN EARLY STAGE CAN PROTECT YOUR HEALTH

If your arteries are getting clogged, you could reduce the risk of a heart attack or stroke, and potentially add healthy years to your life, by slowing or stopping the progression of artery clogging.

This chapter reviews both the well-known health consequences of artery clogging and also some lesser-known consequences.

Because artery clogging is caused by "bad" LDL cholesterol (see chapter 2), preventing further artery clogging by controlling your level of LDL cholesterol could prevent or delay these serious health consequences.

Artery Clogging Can Lead to a Heart Attack, a Stroke, or Vascular Dementia

If the arteries are slowly getting clogged and are left untreated, the plaque in a certain location may eventually burst and then may cause a blood clot that blocks the flow of blood. A blood clot in an artery can result in a heart attack, stroke, or vascular dementia, as the U.S. National Institutes of Health (NIH) has described (see chapter 1).

It is well known that a heart attack can result in death. A stroke may also cause death or may cause brain damage that might require nursing home care. Multiple mini-strokes over time can cause "vascular dementia" (see chapter 1) that cripples brain functions, possibly requiring care from a family member or in an assisted living facility.

Artery Clogging Can Cause Four Other Diseases

As explained by the U.S. National Institutes of Health, artery clogging can also lead to the following:

- peripheral artery disease, which reduces blood flow to the legs and arms, possibly leading to pain while walking, as well as sores, infections, and even death of tissue, called gangrene
- renal artery "stenosis"—that is, artery clogging that limits blood flow to the kidneys, which can

result in high blood pressure or decreased kidney function

- vertebral artery disease, which can limit blood flow to the back of the brain, which "controls body functions that are needed to keep you alive"

- "mesenteric artery ischemia," a disease characterized by reduced blood flow to the intestines that may cause abdominal pain after eating, and diarrhea.

Artery Clogging Can Cause Poor Aging

Artery clogging can also lead to "poor aging due to loss of function in multiple organs" and impaired sexual response, according to a state-of-the-art review article published in the *American Journal of Preventive Cardiology* in 2022.

Early-Stage Artery Clogging Can Slow Down Your Brain

Artery clogging can also slow down the brain, according to a study by 16 researchers published in the *Journal of the American College of Cardiology* in 2021.

The researchers evaluated participants who had early-stage plaque in the carotid arteries that carry blood to the brain. These individuals were found to have "reduced brain metabolism," indicating lower brain activity, relative to participants with unclogged arteries. Areas of the brain showing reduced metabolism included those "known to be affected in dementia."

The researchers pointed to "the need to control cardiovascular risk factors early in life in order to reduce the brain's midlife vulnerability to future cognitive dysfunction."

4

SHOULD YOU GET TESTED
FOR ARTERY CLOGGING?

Five cardiologists (heart doctors) have proposed that people should be tested for artery clogging, in an article published in the *Journal of the American College of Cardiology* in 2019.

They did not recommend, however, who should get tested for artery clogging. (For details on all studies, see the "notes" section at the end of this book.)

Every adult in the U.S. has the choice to get tested for artery clogging (see chapter 5), but there is no clear medical guidance on who should get tested, or when.

Research has shown that unless your level of "bad" LDL cholesterol is relatively low, it is likely that plaque is gradually building up in your arteries, presenting a number of health risks (see chapters 2 and 3).

But if you learn that you have artery clogging, you could consider incorporating additional healthy lifestyle choices if possible, and you could talk with your doctor about starting statin therapy to lower the level of LDL in your blood (see chapters 6 and 7).

Statin therapy can effectively limit further artery clogging and reduce the likelihood of a heart attack, stroke, or other health consequences, potentially adding healthy years to your life.

Fortunately, statin drugs are now generic and therefore inexpensive. All in all, there are good reasons to get tested for artery clogging, even though testing currently requires some time, effort and expense (see chapter 5).

Still, some people have more good reasons to get tested for artery clogging than others.

Until doctors start offering a screening test for artery clogging as part of a regular physical exam, this chapter discusses several factors you could consider in deciding whether to get tested for artery clogging—and if so, whether to get tested soon or to wait a while.

The most important consideration discussed in this chapter may be that testing for artery clogging can identify the value of reducing LDL at a younger age than the "risk scoring" method that doctors currently use to decide whether to recommend statin therapy for any given patient.

This chapter also explores how a screening test may be more likely to find artery clogging in certain individuals: those with a higher level of "bad" LDL cholesterol or higher blood pressure; those with certain other health conditions; those with sub-Saharan or South Asian ancestry; and those with a "low socio-economic status."

For people aged 40-75 with diabetes, this chapter discusses medical guidance that advises statin therapy on that basis alone.

Regrettably, there is no clear guidance on the age at which to begin screening for artery clogging. A case can be made to begin screening in your 40s, in your 50s, or at least by your 60s, as discussed in this chapter.

Ultimately, the choice is yours. Read on for the details.

Testing for Artery Clogging Can Identify the Value of Reducing LDL Earlier than "Risk Scoring" Can

Research has found that testing for artery clogging can be far more accurate than the risk scoring methods widely used by doctors to identify patients who qualify for preventive treatment for artery clogging.

Risk scoring is based on several factors, such as LDL cholesterol level, age, blood pressure, presence or absence of diabetes, and smoking history.

Nineteen researchers have found that a risk scoring method commonly used by U.S. doctors failed to assign intermediate or high risk scores—and thus failed to trigger preventive treatment—in 85% of individuals found to have artery clogging in two or more locations.

Their study was published in the *Journal of the American College of Cardiology* in 2020.

The same research group had previously identified early-stage artery clogging in "nearly 60%" of those classified as having a low risk by traditional risk scoring methods, in a separate study published in the journal *Circulation* in 2015.

Artery Clogging Can Proceed "Unchecked for Decades" Under the Current Risk Scoring Approach

One issue with the risk scoring approach is that it focuses on predicting who will be most likely to have a heart attack or stroke within the next 10 years.

Cardiologists Ann Marie Navar and Eric Peterson have said that "waiting for a person to reach an age when their 10-year predicted cardiovascular risk exceeds a certain arbitrary threshold before recommending a statin allows atherosclerosis to proceed unchecked for decades," in an editorial published in the *Journal of the American Medical Association* in 2022. (Atherosclerosis is the medical term for artery clogging.)

The view of this book's author is that the 10-year time frame considered by the risk scoring method does not serve those of us who want to live longer than 10 more years and also to avoid vascular dementia and other losses of function during our lifetime.

Seven researchers have found that the risk scoring method did not result in adequate statin therapy even for most of those who should have been identified by the method's formula as needing therapy. Analyzing data from the 2015-2016 U.S. National Health and Nutrition Examination Survey, the researchers considered all patients with an estimated 10-year risk of a cardiovascular "event"—such as a heart attack—that was high enough that it should have led to a statin prescription. Of those patients, less than one-third actually took a statin medication. The study was published in the *Journal of the American College of Cardiology* in 2019.

Despite these serious problems with risk scoring, the method does result in treatment for many people with artery clogging.

So if your primary care provider hasn't scored your risk already, you could ask your provider to determine your risk score.

If you receive a statin prescription based on an intermediate or high risk score, and the statin reduces your LDL cholesterol to a level low enough to stop further artery clogging (see chapter 2), you could ask your primary care provider about any future testing for artery clogging. If you are not comfortable taking a prescribed statin medication, however, a screening test that showed artery clogging could inform your decision, as discussed at the end of this chapter.

Five Cardiologists Have Proposed Testing People for Clogged Arteries

As mentioned early in this chapter, five cardiologists have proposed that primary care providers test people for clogged arteries and offer a prescription for "intensive" statin therapy to those found to have the disease, in order to prevent heart attacks and strokes.

Their proposal would overhaul current medical practice.

The cardiologists proposed, as a substitute for the medical profession's risk scoring criteria, to "treat the disease rather than the likelihood of disease" by directly testing for clogged arteries.

Artery clogging that has not yet caused symptoms can be detected, they said, using any of four "readily available" imaging tests that are "noninvasive"—meaning they are performed without so much as a needle prick. These four types of tests are described in chapter 5.

The cardiologists said that most heart attacks occur due to the rupture of plaque on an artery wall, and that plaque progression is "a necessary and modifiable step" between early-stage artery clogging and plaque rupture that can cause a heart attack. The cardiologists reached these conclusions based on their review of prior medical studies.

In patients for whom screening finds early-stage artery clogging, the cardiologists recommended "intensive" lipid-lowering therapy to "halt" the progression of plaque, which "should reduce" the likelihood of a heart attack or stroke, they said.

The cardiologists did not suggest how to determine which patients should be advised to obtain noninvasive screening that checks for artery clogging.

Three Cardiologists Have Called for Screening "At the Earliest Age Possible"

Three cardiologists concluded, based on a review of prior research, that "many" people between the ages of 20 and 50 would benefit from early intervention for artery clogging and that "screening for plaque can be useful" in identifying those who would benefit.

They recommended screening "at the earliest age possible" in an article published in the *American Journal of Preventive Cardiology* in 2022.

The U.S. Preventive Services Task Force Has Made a Compelling Argument for Screening for Artery Clogging

The U.S. Preventive Services Task Force, described on its website as an "independent, volunteer panel of national experts in disease prevention and evidence-based medicine," has made a compelling argument for carotid artery screening.

The task force said that plaque in the carotid arteries, known to doctors as atherosclerosis, "is a manifestation of systemic atherosclerotic [artery-clogging] disease, so identifying this condition may potentially lead to changes in medical management to prevent future cardiovascular events," such as heart attacks and strokes, in a 2021 document called a "final evidence review."

Surprisingly, the task force did not recommend preventing future cardiovascular events in this way, as its members considered in their review only surgical treatment of advanced artery clogging, not healthy choices or statin therapy for early-stage artery clogging.

Seven Cardiologists Have Acknowledged the Possible Value of Detecting Carotid Artery Plaque

Seven doctors who are fellows of the American College of Cardiology said that "carotid plaque detection may provide incremental information" for assessing the risk of cardiovascular disease caused by artery clogging, in a workbook published by the American College of Cardiology in 2022.

For people aged 40-75 with Diabetes, Medical Guidance Advises Statin Therapy on that Basis Alone

Medical guidance from the American College of Cardiology and the American Heart Association published in 2019 recommends moderate-intensity statin therapy for those with diabetes aged 40-75, as well as risk assessment to consider a high-intensity statin.

Although doctors are guided to prescribe a statin to patients in this age group with diabetes, those individuals may still benefit from testing for artery clogging for two reasons.

First, a test for artery clogging may indicate the benefit of intensifying statin therapy beyond the level initially prescribed by the doctor. Second, if an individual is not comfortable taking a pre-scribed statin medication, a screening test that showed artery clogging could help in making that decision, as discussed at the end of this chapter.

The Higher the LDL Level, the More Likely that Screening Will Find Artery Clogging

Among otherwise healthy people with a moderately high level of "bad" LDL cholesterol above 130 mg/dL, most had artery clogging by their mid-40s, as found in a 2018 study discussed in chapter 2.

The results of the study, as shown in the bar chart below, demonstrate that the likelihood of a detectable level of artery clogging increases at higher LDL levels.

Percentage of subjects, most in their 40s, with artery clogging at increasing LDL levels

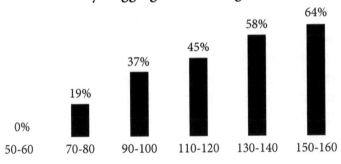

LDL cholesterol level (intermediate data not shown)

The study participants had none of the following four major risk factors for cardiovascular disease: high blood pressure, diabetes, a history of smoking, or a family history of cardiovascular disease.

Screening May Find Artery Clogging
Even in Some People in Their 40s
with a Relatively Low LDL Level

In the same study discussed above, nearly one in five healthy people with a seemingly healthy LDL level of 70-80 mg/dL had artery clogging by their mid-40s.

This is shown on the left side of the bar chart above.

Screening Will More Likely Find
Artery Clogging Among Those
with a Blood Pressure above 130/80

Even a mild form of high blood pressure—where the first number is from 130-139 or the second number is from 80-89—is associated with a higher likelihood of artery clogging, six researchers reported in an article published in the *American Journal of Hypertension* in 2020.

At blood pressure readings above those levels, the researchers found that the prevalence and burden of artery clogging increased. (A reading of 130/80 or above is the current definition of high blood pressure in the U.S.)

After Age 50, Screening May Find Artery Clogging Among Those with a Systolic Blood Pressure Above 120

Among those in their 50s and 60s with a systolic (first number) blood pressure of 120-129, 41% were found to have coronary artery calcium—that is, calcified plaque in their coronary arteries—according to a study by 10 researchers published in the journal *JAMA Cardiology* in 2020.

The Mayo Clinic and Cleveland Clinic Suggest Carotid Artery Ultrasound Testing for Those with High Blood Pressure

The Mayo Clinic health care system says in an article on its website that a doctor "may recommend" a carotid artery ultrasound test for a patient with "a medical condition that increases the risk of a stroke, including high blood pressure."

Similarly, the Cleveland Clinic health care system says on its website that "you may need a carotid ultrasound if you have high blood pressure."

Note that these clinics were likely referring to a full carotid artery ultrasound examination that requires a doctor's order, as described in chapter 5, rather than a carotid artery ultrasound screening test that is available without a doctor's order.

The U.S. Centers for Disease Control Advises How to Measure Your Blood Pressure

Because having an accurate measurement of your blood pressure is valuable for maintaining good health, the U.S. Centers for Disease Control and Prevention has published directions for properly measuring blood pressure, whether in a doctor's office, in a pharmacy with a digital blood pressure measurement machine, or at home with a home blood pressure monitor. The directions are available on the internet at https://www.cdc.gov/bloodpressure/measure.htm

---

Screening May Find Artery Clogging in Blacks at a Younger Age than in Whites

Black Americans had a higher prevalence of strokes than white Americans across all age groups, nine researchers found in an analysis of national health interview data from 619,000 individuals obtained from 2000 to 2009. Black Americans had equivalent prevalence rates for strokes 10 years earlier than whites, the researchers reported, in an article published in the *Journal of Urban Health* in 2016.

Because artery clogging leads to strokes, it is reasonable to expect that Black Americans would also have a higher prevalence of artery clogging than white Americans across all age groups.

Twelve Risk Factors that Indicate
that Screening May Find Artery Clogging

Based on a review of prior research, cardiologist Peter Toth with the CGH Medical Center in Illinois found that coronary artery clogging is more likely among those who have one or more of six risk factors, as reported in an article published in the *American Journal of Preventive Cardiology* in 2020. Those six risk factors are:

- family history of one or more heart attacks or strokes
- male gender
- history of smoking
- diabetes (also see the section above: "For People Aged 40-75 with Diabetes, Medical Guidance Advises Statin Therapy on that Basis Alone")
- persistent inflammatory disease, such as rheumatoid arthritis, psoriasis, HIV or colitis
- sub-Saharan ancestry.

Other "risk enhancers" for artery clogging, noted in medical guidelines published in 2019 by the American College of Cardiology and the American Heart Association, are:

- an LDL level of 160-189 mg/dL
- chronic kidney disease

- metabolic syndrome
- for women, preeclampsia or premature meno-
  pause
- South Asian ancestry.

A study by five researchers found that those with a "low socioeconomic status" were also more likely to have artery clogging, which the researchers identified using a carotid artery ultrasound exam, as reported in an article published in the journal *Atherosclerosis* in 2022.

The researchers identified low socioeconomic status at the neighborhood level based on an index combining measures of deprivation including economic, ethno-racial, age-based, and social marginalization.

Screening is More Likely to Find Artery Clogging Among Those with Obstructive Sleep Apnea

People with obstructive sleep apnea are more likely to have plaque in their coronary arteries, 10 researchers found in a study published in the *American Journal of Preventive Cardiology* in 2023.

Screening is More Likely to Find Artery Clogging Among Men with Erectile Dysfunction

"Erectile dysfunction is a well-established, indepen-dent marker for cardiovascular disease risk," reported a study by 24 researchers published in the *American Journal of Medicine* in 2014.

A Higher Lifetime Exposure to LDL Cholesterol Results in a Greater Risk of a Heart Attack or Stroke

Ten researchers found that a lower LDL level beginning early in life results in a "3-fold greater reduction" in the risk of coronary artery disease than lowering LDL to the same level beginning later in life. In other words, to maintain healthy arteries, a level of "bad" LDL cholesterol that is lower for longer is better.

Looking at this issue from another perspective, 15 researchers reported that cardiovascular disease "event risk," such as a heart attack or stroke, depends on cumulative prior exposure to LDL cholesterol, in a study published in the *Journal of the American College of Cardiology* in 2020.

A Cumulative 5,000 "Milligram-Years" of LDL Exposure "Seems to Be the Tipping Point"

Three cardiologists have explained that the concept of lifetime or cumulative LDL exposure is similar to the concept of lifetime pack-years of smoking. But instead of pack-years, the risk exposure measure for LDL is "milligram-years" of lifetime exposure.

A person with a lifetime average LDL cholesterol level of 125 milligrams per deciliter (mg/dL), they said, will be exposed to a cumulative 5,000 milligram-years of LDL cholesterol by age 40 (because 125 times 40 equals 5,000). That level of exposure "seems to be the tipping point" at which the risk of disease due to artery clogging "starts to increase," they said.

The cardiologists presented this viewpoint in an "expert analysis" article published on the American College of Cardiology's website—not in a peer-reviewed medical journal—in 2018.

If you believe, based on this expert analysis and the peer-reviewed study from 2020 described in the previous section, that cumulative prior exposure to LDL may influence the amount of plaque in the arteries, you could estimate your cumulative prior LDL exposure, which equals your age multiplied by your average lifetime LDL level. If the result is more than 5,000—the value seen by three cardiologists as a "tipping point"—that could suggest a higher likelihood that a screening test would identify artery clogging.

A Reason to Start Screening in Your 40s: Early-Stage Artery Clogging is Common in Middle Age

Artery clogging progressed "significantly" in 41% of a group of 3,514 apparently healthy middle-aged men and women over a three-year period, 13 researchers found in a study published in the *Journal of the American College of Cardiology* in 2020.

The progression of artery clogging is linked to heart attacks and strokes, the authors said, citing earlier research.

Even in individuals seen as having a low risk of heart disease, progression of artery clogging was found in 36% of study participants.

Progression was measured both as an increase in the number of locations at which arterial plaque was found, and as an increase in the total volume of arterial plaque.

A Reason to Start Screening in Your 40s or 50s: Guidance from Screening Providers

The company Life Line Screening, which provides carotid artery ultrasound screening tests, says that such screening "is appropriate" for adults aged 55 and older, and also for adults aged 40 and older "who have risk factors for cardiovascular disease, and who want to be proactive about their health."

The Heart Health Foundation offers free artery screenings in two states for those 50 and older who have at least one of these risk factors: a history of smoking, diabetes, high blood pressure, high cholesterol, or a family history of heart disease. (As noted earlier in this chapter, medical guidance advises statin therapy for those aged 40-75 with diabetes.)

A Reason for Screening in Your 60s and Older: Artery Clogging is Widespread in that Age Range

Among people aged 60 or older, over 90% of both men and women were considered "positive" for artery clogging based on a positive result from at least one of four different tests, in a study by eight researchers published in the journal *Atherosclerosis* in 2011.

As an indicator from an artery screening service provider, the Heart Health Foundation offers free artery screenings for anyone over 60 years old.

Some Cardiologists Advise Screening as Early as Possible

As discussed earlier in this chapter, three cardiologists have said that screening for plaque can be "useful" for many people aged 20 to 50 to identify those who would benefit from early intervention for artery clogging. They recommended screening "at the earliest age possible."

Perhaps Get Screened if You are Not Comfortable Taking a Prescribed Statin Medication

Some people who have been offered a statin prescription—for instance, because they have an elevated risk of a heart attack or stroke in the next 10 years—may not feel totally comfortable taking the medication as prescribed. They may feel this way even though statins have been found to be generally safe (see chapter 8).

If that sounds like you, you could obtain a carotid artery ultrasound artery screening test to learn whether your arteries are getting clogged. If the results show artery clogging, that could inform your decision on whether to take the statin as prescribed.

As evidence for this possibility, patients who learned that their coronary arteries were getting clogged had a "significantly increased" likelihood of starting or continuing preventive treatment and lifestyle changes compared to patients who saw no evidence of coronary artery clogging, as reported in a study by 13 researchers published in the journal *JACC Cardiovascular Imaging* in 2017.

5

HOW TO GET TESTED
FOR ARTERY CLOGGING

If you've decided to find out whether your arteries are getting clogged, perhaps after reviewing chapter 4 that is intended to help inform such a decision, this chapter describes two options.

Both options use ultrasound technology to detect artery-clogging plaque in the carotid arteries that deliver blood to the brain. Five cardiologists have recommended carotid ultrasound technology as one of four means to detect early-stage artery clogging.

There are two types of carotid artery ultrasound testing: a carotid artery ultrasound screening test, which is the focus of this chapter; and a full carotid artery ultrasound examination, which is discussed at the end of the chapter.

In case a carotid artery ultrasound screening test identifies plaque in your arteries, this chapter discusses the option of sharing the results with your primary care provider and/or with a medical specialist, so you may discuss healthy choices, whether a statin prescription is appropriate, or whether further testing may be desirable.

The information in chapter 2, about the health effects of various levels of "bad" LDL cholesterol, can inform any doctor–patient discussion about the target level of LDL to be reached, whether statin medication may be needed to achieve that target, and if so, the appropriate statin dosage.

To provide context to evaluate the option of getting a carotid artery ultrasound screening test, the final sections of this chapter discuss the option of a full carotid artery examination, as well as three other types of tests to detect artery clogging recommended by the five cardiologists mentioned above. (For further details on the information provided in this chapter, see the "notes" section at the end of this book.)

The Carotid Artery Ultrasound Screening Test

The carotid artery ultrasound screening test is just like the ultrasound test used for pregnant women but is performed on the neck, where the carotid arteries are, instead of the belly. Unlike a medical X-ray or CT scan, an ultrasound test does not involve ionizing radiation and is therefore very safe.

An ultrasound screening test of the carotid arteries on both sides of the neck is widely available in the U.S. without a doctor's order, and can be performed in as little as five minutes.

The other types of tests recommended by the five cardiologists all require a doctor's order.

The carotid artery ultrasound screening test estimates the amount of plaque in each carotid artery based largely on the speed of blood flow through the artery as identified by ultrasound technology. The speed of blood flow indicates the extent of artery clogging because an artery with some plaque is narrower than a healthy artery without plaque, and so a given amount of blood entering the artery with plaque must flow faster to pass through it.

Carotid artery ultrasound screening is not yet routinely available to patients at their doctor's office.

Several Providers in the U.S. Offer Carotid Artery Screening without a Doctor's Order

At least three service providers and one health care system in the U.S. offer carotid artery ultrasound screening without a doctor's order and inform screening participants whether they have early-stage artery clogging.

Recognizing the value of carotid artery ultrasound screening, about 40 other U.S. health care systems across 24 states also offer the screening, but unfortunately, they have not disclosed whether they inform screening participants when they discover early-stage artery clogging, or only when they discover advanced artery clogging.

Life Line Screening offers screening at locations nationwide: The company Life Line Screening offers carotid artery ultrasound screening at one-day sessions held across the U.S., offering these "pop-up" screenings at houses of worship, hotels, and community centers.

Life Line Screening provides its customers with a screening result for each carotid artery stating whether the artery is free of plaque or has mild, moderate, or severe clogging. The "mild" and "moderate" categories indicate earlier-stage artery clogging.

The company offers a carotid artery ultrasound screening test for $85 and schedules appointments through its website or by phone.

As one point for comparison, the author of this book obtained a screening test from this company after receiving a comprehensive carotid artery ultrasound exam from the health care system Johns Hopkins Medicine, which a preventive cardiologist interpreted as showing a 30% to 40% narrowing in one of the carotid arteries due to plaque. The author's Life Line Screening carotid artery ultrasound screening test, obtained after the comprehensive carotid artery exam, also identified "mild" early-stage clogging in that artery.

The Heart Health Foundation offers screening in two states: The foundation offers free carotid artery ultrasound screening in Maryland and North Carolina for those who meet its eligibility requirements, through its Dare to CARE program.

The foundation provides a screening result for each carotid artery stating whether the artery is free of plaque or has some level of clogging. The "mild" and "moderate" levels of clogging indicate artery blockage of 1% to 59%.

The foundation provides appointment scheduling information on its website.

Health Gauge Screenings offers screening in the Midwest: The company Health Gauge Screenings, based in Des Moines, Iowa, offers carotid artery ultrasound screening in combination with other screening tests for $185. Screening results show whether each carotid artery is free of plaque, has mild or moderate clogging up to 50%, or has significant or "critical" clogging.

Atrium Health Navicent offers screening in Georgia: The screening program offered by health care system Atrium Health Navicent incorporates the use of a contrast dye injected into the blood. This enables the inclusion of high-contrast ultrasound images in the patient report that are easy for a doctor to interpret, while adding a layer of complication.

The screening report shows the extent of carotid artery blockage in one of two categories: blockage of zero to 50%, and blockage of 50% or more. For those found to have a blockage of zero to 50%, the report provides additional information that a doctor, a cardiologist, or a preventive cardiologist may be willing to interpret to determine whether there is any artery clogging and if so, how much. The screening costs $50; the screening program provides scheduling information on its web page.

About 40 health care systems offer screening but may not report early-stage artery clogging: The rest of the approximately 40 U.S. health care systems that offer carotid artery ultrasound screening, which were identified through an internet search, have not publicly disclosed whether they report early-stage artery clogging to screening participants, or only late-stage clogging.

For example, a report of zero to 50% artery clogging might mean zero artery clogging or it might mean 49% artery clogging. Without additional information indicating where one stands in that range of zero to 50%, such a report would not indicate whether the individual has early-stage artery clogging.

That matters because a report of early-stage clogging can prompt early action to protect one's health, as discussed in chapters 3, 4, 6 and 7.

Because many health care systems offer surgical options for those with late-stage artery clogging, it is possible that some of these health care systems that offer screening are focused on identifying people who could benefit from artery surgery, also known as vascular surgery.

Any of these health care systems may be willing to disclose to an individual prospective screening participant whether they report early-stage artery clogging, even though they have not disclosed this information on their website. The health care systems that offer carotid artery ultrasound screening may be identified through an internet search.

Some surgery centers offer carotid artery ultrasound screening: Some medical practices that perform artery surgery, or vascular surgery, also provide artery screening, in part to help identify patients with advanced artery clogging who may be eligible for surgery. Because these practices focus on surgery rather than on preventing further artery clogging through healthy choices and/or statin therapy—the focus of this book—their artery screening offerings are not discussed here.

Some other providers offer a "CIMT" test: Some other providers offer a different type of carotid artery test known as a carotid intima-media thickness test, or CIMT test. This test measures the width of a carotid artery's wall. While an increased width of the artery wall may indicate a decline in the artery's health even before plaque forms on the inside of the artery wall, this book does not further discuss the CIMT test for two reasons. First, of the four studies discussing CIMT that are referenced in the American College of Cardiology workbook discussed in chapter 4, the two most recent studies both found that the presence of carotid plaque is a better predictor of future heart attacks and strokes than the width of the carotid artery's wall. Second, there has been limited discussion in the recent medical literature about using the results of a CIMT test to guide statin therapy or other treatment decisions.

The Availability of Carotid Artery Screening May Improve Over Time

The number of screening providers that provide results assessing early-stage artery clogging may increase over time, as the value of artery screening becomes more widely known.

In the future, more of the approximately 40 health care systems offering carotid artery ultrasound screening may publicly disclose the type of information they provide to screening participants, and for some of those health care systems, the information provided may indicate whether the screening participant has early-stage artery clogging. In that case, those health care systems would become good choices for carotid artery ultrasound screening.

The availability of screening may also improve because any medical doctor may purchase handheld ultrasound equipment at a relatively low cost and begin offering ultrasound artery screening to their patients. The American College of Emergency Physicians issued a policy statement in 2018 concluding that handheld ultrasound devices, when used by trained physicians, produce images "comparable" to those produced with the use of traditional, more costly ultrasound machines. At least eight different brands of handheld ultrasound devices are available, according to an article published in the journal *Current Emergency and Hospital Medicine Reports* in 2021.

Next Steps if a Screening Test Shows that Your Arteries Have Plaque

An artery screening test that identifies plaque in either or both of the carotid arteries also suggests that plaque may exist in other arteries throughout the body.

If a carotid artery ultrasound screening test shows your carotid arteries have plaque, you may discuss the results with your primary care provider or a cardiologist. You may discuss healthy choices and ask whether a statin prescription would be appropriate for you.

No doctor would consider offering a statin prescription without some medical basis, and many doctors would consider evidence of plaque in your arteries to be relevant medical information.

Another option, if you'd like, would be to request an appointment with a preventive cardiologist to discuss your results with them, either as your initial discussion or as a second opinion (see chapter 9).

Before an appointment, you could review the early sections of chapter 2 that discuss research findings that can inform a target level of "bad" LDL cholesterol for those who have plaque in their arteries.

During an appointment, a primary care provider, cardiologist, or preventive cardiologist looking at carotid artery ultrasound screening test results might decide to order a full carotid artery ultrasound exam, which provides more information than a carotid artery ultrasound screening test. The full carotid artery ultrasound exam is more extensive, takes longer, and is therefore more expensive, but the cost may be covered by insurance.

Next Steps if a Screening Test Does *Not* Indicate that Your Arteries Have Plaque

Just as there is no medical guidance on who should get screened for artery clogging or when to get screened, there is no medical guidance on when to get a follow-up screening if the first screening does not identify artery clogging. Here again, each of us is on our own to make that decision.

If the ultrasound artery screening test becomes more sensitive at some point and is able to detect plaque at an earlier stage, that could be a good time to schedule another screening test.

One program that offers free artery screenings has offered to each participant who receives a "normal" result—indicating no plaque—a free follow-up screening in five years.

A Full Carotid Artery Ultrasound Exam (Not a Screening Test) Requires a Doctor's Order

Some doctors may be willing to order a full carotid artery ultrasound artery exam, which is more extensive than a screening test, perhaps on the basis of a high blood pressure reading (see chapter 4) or some other reason, to identify the presence and extent of any plaque in the arteries.

Such an exam takes about 20 minutes and costs more than a screening test, but the cost may be covered by insurance. If you'd like to pursue this possibility, a preventive cardiologist may be more willing to consider the request than a primary care provider or a traditional cardiologist (see chapter 9).

Three Other Types of Artery Tests Recommended by Five Cardiologists

This chapter does not focus on the other three types of tests recommended by the five cardiologists who recommended screening people for early-stage artery clogging—as discussed in chapter 4—because the other tests are not widely available from a service provider without a doctor's order.

One of the three other tests is an ultrasound scan of a major artery below the kidneys known as the infrarenal aorta. The other two are versions of a coronary artery calcium (CAC) test that assesses the level of calcium in the coronary arteries that bring oxygenated blood to the heart muscle. Both versions of the CAC test use a type of X-ray called computed tomography; one version uses a contrast agent, while the other does not.

A full carotid artery ultrasound exam, discussed in the previous section, has been found to be superior to a CAC test for detecting early-stage artery clogging, in a study by 14 researchers published in the *Journal of the American College of Cardiology* in 2021. That makes sense because "calcification" of an artery—meaning the addition of calcium to the plaque in an artery—"is traditionally a later-stage manifestation" of artery clogging, as three cardiologists reported in an article published in the journal *Atherosclerosis* in 2022.

6

IF YOU HAVE ARTERY CLOGGING: HEALTHY CHOICES

There are two ways to protect the health of your arteries: healthy lifestyle changes and medication, typically a statin medication. This chapter and the next discuss these options.

Healthy lifestyle changes, although they can be difficult to make, can be quite effective in reducing the level of "bad" LDL cholesterol, which causes artery clogging.

The American Heart Association promotes eight healthy habits: eat better, be more active, quit tobacco, get healthy sleep, manage weight, control cholesterol, manage blood sugar, and manage blood pressure.

The first recommendation on that list—basically, a healthy diet—is the focus of this chapter. The other seven recommendations are fairly straightforward.

But when it comes to a healthy diet, the choices can be confusing because so many health claims are made about so many various diets.

This chapter focuses on dietary recommendations published in the *American Journal of Preventive Cardiology* and dietary guidance from the American Heart Association.

Preventive Cardiologists Recommend Four Diets: Mediterranean, "DASH," "Healthy Vegetarian," and Vegan

The "optimal" diet to prevent artery clogging, and thus avoid cardiovascular disease, consists predominantly of "fruits, vegetables, legumes, nuts, seeds, plant protein and fatty fish," said a team of preventive cardiologists—heart doctors with a focus on prevention—and other researchers. They reached that conclusion in an article based on their review of prior research, published in the *American Journal of Preventive Cardiology* in 2022. (For details on all studies, see the "notes" section at the end of this book.)

The 14 researchers said that four diets meet guidelines issued in 2019 that were similar to their "optimal" diet recommendations: the Mediterranean diet, the "DASH" diet, a "healthy vegetarian" diet, and the exclusively plant-based, or vegan, diet.

The authors' recommendations were based on their review of 172 research studies and constitute a "clinical practice statement" from the American Society for Preventive Cardiology.

One category of recommended foods—legumes—includes beans, peas and peanuts. Another category—seeds—includes foods such as wheat (from which bread is made), rice, oats, and nuts.

The 14 co-authors advised reducing the consumption of foods containing saturated fat, dietary cholesterol, salt, and refined grain, as well as ultra-processed foods.

Foods with saturated fat include eggs, meats, whole milk, butter, and coconut oil. Dietary cholesterol is found in meats, seafood, poultry, eggs, and dairy products. The most commonly used refined grain is white flour, which is used to make white bread. White flour is made by removing the outer bran and the "wheat germ" from wheat seeds, before milling the seeds into flour.

Ultra-processed food includes calorie-dense foods high in refined flour, sugar and/or fats, such as snacks, treats and many fast food and restaurant offerings. In a separate study, six researchers found that ultra-processed foods were the source of 58% of the calories consumed in America, as reported in an article published in the journal *BMJ Open* in 2016.

For those interested in a vegan diet, the Academy of Nutrition and Dietetics has noted that "vegans need reliable sources of vitamin B-12, such as fortified foods or supplements," in a position statement published in the *Journal of the Academy of Nutrition and Dietetics* in 2016.

The American Heart Association Favors Mediterranean, DASH-style, and Mostly Vegetarian Diets

The American Heart Association (AHA) favors Mediterranean, DASH-style, and mostly vegetarian diets that include eggs and milk, and that may include fish as well, the association said in a scientific statement that compared various diets to the AHA's dietary guidance, and that was published in the journal *Circulation* in 2023. The AHA categorized all these diets as "Tier 1" diets.

Slightly less favored by the AHA are vegan diets and low-fat diets, which the association categorized as "Tier 2" diets.

The statement said that very-low-fat diets and low-carbohydrate diets have "low to moderate alignment" with AHA dietary guidance, categorizing them as "Tier 3" diets.

Paleo and ketogenic diets "align poorly" with AHA dietary guidance, the association said, categorizing these diets as "Tier 4" diets.

7

IF YOU HAVE ARTERY CLOGGING: STATIN THERAPY

If an ultrasound screening test shows you have artery clogging, you may discuss the test results with your primary care provider, a cardiologist (heart doctor) or a preventive cardiologist, and you may ask about statin therapy to reduce your level of "bad" LDL cholesterol. (LDL cholesterol causes artery clogging, as discussed in chapter 2.)

Statin therapy can prevent a heart attack by stabilizing existing artery-clogging plaque. It can also slow, stop, or potentially reverse artery clogging. This chapter focuses on these benefits.

Many primary care providers and cardiologists discuss statin therapy with a patient with a "shared decision-making" frame of mind. Perhaps the idea is to reach a medical recommendation that the patient accepts, given that every patient chooses whether to fill any prescription and take the medication prescribed.

So if you are about to enter that conversation with a primary care provider or cardiologist, you could consider several factors that affect your health:

- the level of LDL cholesterol in your blood, as shown in your most recent blood test known as a "lipid panel"
- the health effects of various levels of LDL cholesterol, as discussed in chapter 2
- the ability of statin therapy to stabilize artery-clogging plaque and to slow, stop, or even reverse plaque progression, discussed below
- the effectiveness of various levels of statin therapy, also discussed below
- statin safety, as discussed in chapter 8.

Statin Therapy Can Prevent a Heart Attack by Stabilizing Existing Artery-Clogging Plaque

Statin drugs stabilize "vulnerable" plaques in the arteries, reducing the likelihood that a plaque will rupture and cause a clot that can slow or stop the flow of blood, as reported in a study by five cardiologists. The authors reported that the majority of "coronary artery events"— that is, heart attacks—occur as a result of plaque rupture.

In other words, preventing plaque rupture by stabilizing plaque can prevent heart attacks.

The study, based on a review of prior medical research, was published in the *Journal of the American College of Cardiology* in 2019. (For details on all studies, see the "notes" section at the end of this book.)

Statin Therapy Can Slow, Stop, or Reverse Plaque Progression

The same five cardiologists mentioned above concluded that "intensive" lipid-lowering therapy such as statin therapy can "halt" the progression of plaque, which "should reduce" the likelihood of a heart attack or stroke. They reached this conclusion through a review of prior medical research, in the same article mentioned immediately above.

A study by 26 researchers found that artery-clogging plaque regressed in study participants whose LDL level was reduced to 70 mg/dL or below. Artery blockage due to plaque, measured as a percentage of the artery's cross-section, regressed by up to two percentage points within the first year. The study, published in the *Journal of the American College of Cardiology* in 2015, is described in chapter 2.

Eleven researchers found "significant reductions" in a plaque component known as "lipid-rich necrotic core" after one year of statin therapy, in a study published in the *Journal of Neuroradiology* in 2017.

Effectiveness of Various Levels of Statin Therapy

The dosage of any statin medication is classified as "high-intensity" if it reduces "bad" LDL cholesterol by at least 50% on average. The dosage is classified as "moderate-intensity" if it reduces LDL cholesterol by 30% to 50% on average. These definitions are from guidelines for management of elevated cholesterol prepared jointly by the European Society of Cardiology and the European Atherosclerosis Society and published in the *European Heart Journal* in 2020.

This information may be useful in any discussion with a primary care provider or cardiologist about statin dosage, especially if you know your current level of "bad" LDL cholesterol and you have a target level of LDL cholesterol in mind—perhaps based on the medical findings about various LDL levels presented in chapter 2.

For those at the greatest risk of a heart attack or stroke, a doctor may prescribe a newer nonstatin LDL-lowering medication, perhaps in combination with a statin drug.

8

HOW SAFE ARE STATINS?

This chapter presents the guidance on statin safety prepared jointly by the American College of Cardiology and the American Heart Association, as well as the statin safety guidance of the European Society of Cardiology, and additional guidance from the Mayo Clinic health care system.

Statin Therapy is Usually Well Tolerated and Safe, Says the American Guideline

Side effects from statins are "infrequent or rare" in clinical trials, and statin therapy is "usually well tolerated and safe," according to the guideline on cholesterol management jointly issued by the American College of Cardiology (ACC) and the American Heart Association (AHA). The guideline was published in the *Journal of the American College of Cardiology* in 2019. (For details on all journal articles, see the "notes" section at the end of this book.)

The most frequent statin-associated side effects, the guideline says, are muscle symptoms, usually muscle pain, reported in 5% to 20% of patients.

Statins "modestly" increase the risk of diabetes among those who have risk factors for diabetes, "but this should not be cause for discontinuation," the guideline says. Liver problems are infrequent, while the medical condition known as rhabdomyolysis is rare, as are other side effects, the guideline adds.

Rhabdomyolysis is potentially fatal, according to the U.S. Centers for Disease Control.

The Mayo Clinic health care system states that rhabdomyolysis or milder forms of muscle inflammation from statins can be diagnosed with a blood test measuring the level of the enzyme creatine kinase. The Mayo Clinic advises in a website post addressed to patients that "if you notice moderate or severe muscle aches after starting to take a statin, contact your doctor."

The ACC/AHA guideline says that a primary care provider prescribing a statin should assess the patient's "appropriate safety indicators" sometime between 4 and 12 weeks after starting a statin or adjusting the dose, and also review the patient's adherence to any recommended lifestyle changes and the patient's LDL cholesterol level. Assessments should be repeated every 3 to 12 months, the guideline says, based on the need to assess adherence or safety.

The ACC/AHA guideline says there is "no definite association" between statin therapy and cancer.

The guideline's table 11 provides more detail on side effects.

Among those who experience side effects, the guideline says that the "large majority" are able to tolerate an alternative statin or an alternative regimen, such as a reduced dose, or a reduced dose in combination with a nonstatin cholesterol-lowering drug.

The ACC/AHA guideline recommends a doctor-patient risk discussion before starting statin therapy, to weigh the potential for reducing the risk of cardiovascular disease against the potential for statin-associated side effects and statin–drug interactions. In this discussion, the guideline says the primary care provider should emphasize that "side effects can be addressed successfully."

Adverse Effects of Statins are Rare, Says the European Guideline

Adverse effects of statin therapy are rare, says the European Society of Cardiology (ESC) in its guideline on cardiovascular disease prevention, published in the

European Heart Journal in 2021. The most frequent adverse effect of statin therapy, the guideline says, is myopathy, a muscle disorder, "but this is rare." (For context, the primary symptom of myopathy is muscle weakness, according to the health care system Penn Medicine, while the American ACC/AHA guideline says the most common muscle symptom is muscle pain.)

The ESC guideline says that the most serious adverse effect, rhabdomyolysis, is "extremely rare."

Increased blood sugar levels that increase the risk of diabetes can occur after statin treatment begins and are "dose dependent, in part linked to slight weight gain," says the ESC guideline, adding that the benefits of statins "outweigh the risks for the majority of patients."

9

WHEN TO SEEK OUT
A PREVENTIVE CARDIOLOGIST

If your arteries are getting clogged, as identified by a carotid artery ultrasound screening test (see chapter 5), and you want a prescription for a statin medication, your primary care provider may be willing to provide that prescription. If you want a statin prescription but your doctor does not offer you one, you could review the following section on working with a preventive cardiologist (a heart doctor who focuses on prevention).

If your primary care provider does offer you a statin prescription, you could follow up, after you've been taking the statin for a while, with a blood test known as a cholesterol panel or "lipid panel" to see your new level of "bad" LDL cholesterol.

Your primary care provider can order a lipid panel, and some medical testing services such as Quest or

LabCorp may offer a lipid panel in your state without a doctor's order.

If you have a target LDL level—perhaps based on the information provided in chapter 2—and your LDL level remains above that target level, you could discuss with your primary care provider the possibility of a higher intensity of statin therapy—that is, a higher dosage. Many primary care providers, however, may not be comfortable offering a statin prescription at a dosage high enough to help you aggressively lower your LDL level. That's where a preventive cardiologist could be helpful in finding an appropriate level of statin medication for you.

Advantages of Working with a Preventive Cardiologist

As the name suggests, a preventive cardiologist focuses on preventing the progression of disease. (In contrast, heart doctors known as interventional cardiologists "intervene" to surgically treat advanced stages of artery disease.)

Preventive cardiologists should be familiar with the medical research described in this book, which has shown the health benefits of aggressively reducing the level of LDL cholesterol so it is low enough to stop further artery clogging.

If a carotid artery ultrasound screening test shows that your arteries are getting clogged, a preventive cardiologist can prescribe statins at a dose high enough to aggressively lower your level of "bad" LDL cholesterol, giving you the greatest chance for healthy arteries that could add healthy years to your life.

How to Find a Preventive Cardiologist

The easiest way to find a preventive cardiologist is to receive a referral from your primary care provider. Yet if that approach does not work, or leads to an unsatisfactory outcome, there are other ways as well.

The appendix that follows this chapter provides a directory of health care systems and medical practices where preventive cardiologists work. The directory may be a useful starting point in locating a preventive cardiologist with whom you feel comfortable.

The appendix also offers suggestions for searching online to identify additional preventive cardiologists beyond those who may be found through the directory, including those who may work at a medical office or health care system closer to where you live.

How to Make your Case when Contacting Preventive Cardiologists

Once you have a list of preventive cardiologists, you may choose to find out which of them is most willing to see you as a patient.

Preventive cardiologists may typically get referrals from primary care providers, and some may not be interested in working with a patient who is searching for a preventive cardiologist on their own. Thus, approaching several preventive cardiologists at once may be the most effective strategy.

Ideally, you do not want to make an appointment with a preventive cardiologist who will end up deciding at your appointment that they are not interested in helping you. It would be better to find out in advance which preventive cardiologist on your list is most interested in working with you.

It may be most effective to make your case either in writing, by email or mail, or briefly over the phone to each preventive cardiologist's scheduler, until you find a preventive cardiologist who you believe will be most helpful to you, and then set an appointment with that provider.

If you decide to take this approach, you could make your case by stating your age; your LDL cholesterol level; any personal and/or family history of heart attacks, strokes, or vascular dementia; any other risk factors (see chapter 4); any results from a carotid artery ultrasound screening test; any symptoms that concern you about the health of your heart and blood vessels—that is, your cardiovascular health; and your treatment goals.

If you would like to contact preventive cardiologists by email, you may need to call each preventive cardiologist's office to request the appropriate email address to use.

Cardiologists who are not accepting new patients may simply not respond to detailed information about your health concern. If you do not receive any satisfactory responses, you could contact preventive cardiologists whose offices are located farther away.

APPENDIX:
DIRECTORY OF PREVENTIVE
CARDIOLOGISTS IN THE U.S.

You may choose to work with a preventive cardiologist—a heart doctor with a focus on prevention—for any of the reasons discussed in chapter 9. If
you would like to work with a preventive cardiologist,
chapter 9 also describes the following:

- how a primary care provider may provide a
  referral to a preventive cardiologist
- how to advocate for yourself if you are searching
  for a preventive cardiologist on your own
- how to identify a preventive cardiologist who is
  most likely to be helpful to you.

The directory in this appendix is designed to help
you search for preventive cardiologists who work in or
near your state. The directory includes health care systems in the U.S. affiliated with a medical school, and

other health providers whose websites enable you to search for a preventive cardiologist.

The directory is a partial list. It does not include health providers that may have preventive cardiologists on staff but do not enable you to search for one on their website. The directory most likely misses a number of small medical practices where preventive cardiologists work.

Because the directory is just a starting point, and unfortunately does not point to preventive cardiologists in every part of the U.S., the section below provides suggestions for searching beyond the providers included in the directory.

Searching Beyond the Directory

If you would like to search for preventive cardiologists not represented in the directory below, this section describes three ways to do so.

First, if your primary care provider is supportive of your interest in preserving the health of your arteries, and understands that a preventive cardiologist is more likely than a traditional cardiologist to work with you toward that goal, you may request a referral from your primary care provider to a preventive cardiologist.

Second, you may search at Google.com, for example by using one of the following phrases:

- preventive cardiologists near me
- preventive cardiologists at [name of nearby hospital or health system]
- preventive cardiologists in [name of your city, a city near you, or your state or a nearby state]

Third, because preventive cardiology is still a relatively new medical specialty and is taught at some medical schools, a hospital near you that is affiliated with a medical school, also known as a teaching hospital, may be the closest location to find a preventive cardiologist. If the teaching hospital closest to you is not already shown in the directory below, you may search on the internet for its website. From that website, you may access the list of cardiologists affiliated with the hospital. You may search that list for the word "preventive" or simply the text "prevent." You could repeat the process for additional teaching hospitals farther away.

The following directory is in alphabetical order by state.

ARIZONA

Phoenix/ Scottsdale: Mayo Clinic

1. Go to the web page: https://www.mayoclinic.org/diseases-conditions/heart-disease/doctors-departments/ddc-20353127

2. Scroll down to just below the phrase "Doctors who treat this condition" and look below the phrase "By location"
3. Select "Phoenix/Scottsdale, AZ
4. Use your computer keyboard's search function to search for: prevent
5. Make a list of all doctors with "prevent" in their description
6. Scroll to the bottom of the list of doctors and advance to the next page of doctors
7. Repeat steps 4 through 6 until you have searched all results pages.

CALIFORNIA

Los Angeles: Cedars Sinai Preventive and Consultative Heart Center

Website: https://www.cedars-sinai.org/programs/heart/specialties/general-cardiology/prevention.html

Phone: 800-CEDARS-1

Orange County: UCI Health / Preventive Cardiology & Cholesterol Management

Website: https://www.ucihealth.org/medical-services/cardiology/preventive-cardiology/

Phone: 714-456-6699

Stanford: Stanford Medicine Health Care, Preventive Cardiology

Website: https://stanfordhealthcare.org/medical-clinics/preventive-cardiology.html

Phone: 650-725-5909

COLORADO

Several locations in Colorado: UC Health

1. Go to the web page: https://www.uchealth.org/provider/
2. In the text box, enter "cardiology" and then under "Areas of Care," select "Cardiology"
3. Choose "Show 50 results per page"
4. Use your computer keyboard's search function to search for: prevent
5. Make a list of all doctors with "prevent" in their description
6. Scroll to the bottom of the page and advance to the next page of results.
7. Repeat steps 4 through 6 until you have searched all results pages.

FLORIDA

Boca Raton: Boca Raton Regional Hospital, Jean and David Blechman Center for Women's Specialty Care and Preventive Cardiology

Website: https://www.brrh.com/Services/Lynn -Womens-Institute/Specialty-Care-Preventive -Cardiology.aspx

Jacksonville: Mayo Clinic

1. Go to the web page: https://www.mayoclinic .org/diseases-conditions/heart-disease/doctors -departments/ddc-20353127
2. Scroll down to just below the phrase "Doctors who treat this condition" and look below the phrase "By location"
3. Select "Jacksonville, FL"
4. Use your computer keyboard's search function to search for: prevent
5. Make a list of all doctors with "prevent" in their description
6. Scroll to the bottom of the list of doctors and advance to the next page of doctors
7. Repeat steps 4 through 6 until you have searched all results pages.

Miami area: University of Miami Health System

1. Go to the web page: https://doctors.umiami health.org

2.   In the search box, enter: cardiology

3.   Under "Specialties," click "Preventive Cardiology"

GEORGIA

Atlanta and northern Georgia: Emory Healthcare

1.   Go to the web page: https://www.emoryhealth care.org/physician-finder/index.html

2.   In the search box under "Need help finding a provider?" enter: cardiology

3.   On the results page, in the box at left labeled "Specialties," select "Preventive Cardiology"

Several locations: Georgia Heart Institute, Center for Cardiovascular Prevention, Metabolism and Lipids

Website: https://www.nghs.com/heart/prevention -center-services/

Phone: 678-675-0794

ILLINOIS

Chicago area: UChicago Medicine

1.   Go to the web page: https://www.uchicago medicine.org/find-a-physician/

2.   Under "Find a Doctor," in the box labeled "Start Your Search," enter: preventive

3. Under the heading "Areas of Expertise," select "Preventive Cardiology"
4. Click on the search box at right.

Chicago area: Northwestern Medicine

1. Go to the web page: https://www.nm.org /doctors
2. In the search box, type but do not enter: cardiology
3. From the drop-down list, select: "Preventive Cardiology"

KENTUCKY

Louisville area: UofL Health

1. Go to the web page: https://uoflhealth.org /providers/
2. In the drop-down box "By Specialty or Service Offered," select "Preventative Cardiology"

MARYLAND

Baltimore and one other location: Johns Hopkins Medicine Heart and Vascular Institute / Ciccarone Center

Website: https://www.hopkinsmedicine.org/heart -vascular-institute/cardiology/ciccarone

Phone: 443-997-0270

MASSACHUSETTS

Boston: Mass General Brigham, Cardiovascular Disease Prevention Center

Website: https://www.massgeneral.org/heart-center
/treatments-and-services/cardiovascular-disease
-prevention/

Phone: 617-726-1843

MINNESOTA

Rochester: Mayo Clinic

1. Go to the web page: https://www.mayoclinic
   .org/diseases-conditions/heart-disease/doctors
   -departments/ddc-20353127

2. Scroll down to just below the phrase "Doctors
   who treat this condition" and look below the
   phrase "By location"

3. Select "Rochester, MN"

4. Use your computer keyboard's search function
   to search for: prevent

5. Make a list of all doctors with "prevent" in their
   description

6. Scroll to the bottom of the list of doctors and
   advance to the next page of doctors.

7. Repeat steps 4 through 6 until you have searched
   all results pages.

NEW JERSEY

Cherry Hill and other locations in New Jersey and Pennsylvania: Penn Medicine

Website: https://www.pennmedicine.org/for-patients-and-visitors/find-a-program-or-service/heart-and-vascular/preventive-cardiovascular/treatment-teams/

Phone: 800-789-7366

NEW YORK

New York City: NYU Langone Health, Center for the Prevention of Cardiovascular Disease

Website: https://nyulangone.org/locations/center-for-the-prevention-of-cardiovascular-disease

Phone: 212-263-0855

New York City metropolitan area: Northwell Health, Center for Heart Disease Prevention and Advanced Lipid Disorders

Website: https://www.northwell.edu/cardiovascular-thoracic-services/find-care/treatments/heart-disease-prevention/

Phone: (855) HEART-11

Suffolk County: Suffolk Heart Group, Heart Attack Prevention Program

Website: https://www.suffolkheartgroup.com/heart-attack-prevention-program/

OKLAHOMA

Tulsa and other locations: Oklahoma Heart Institute

Website: https://oklahomaheart.com/specialty/noninvasive-cardiology/

Phone: 918-592-0999

OREGON

Portland and other locations: OHSU

1. Go to the web page: https://www.ohsu.edu/health/find-a-doctor
2. Type but do not enter in the search box under "Find a Doctor at OHSU": cardiology
3. In the box that appears, under "Conditions and treatments," select "preventative cardiology"

PENNSYLVANIA

Philadelphia and other locations: Temple Health, Preventive Cardiology & Integrative Heart Health Program

Website: https://www.templehealth.org/services/heart-vascular/patient-care/programs/preventive-cardiology-integrative-heart-health

Phone: 800-TEMPLE-MED

Philadelphia and other locations in Pennsylvania and New Jersey: Penn Medicine

Website: https://www.pennmedicine.org/for-patients -and-visitors/find-a-program-or-service/heart-and -vascular/preventive-cardiovascular/treatment-teams/

Phone: 800-789-7366

TEXAS

Dallas / Fort Worth: UT Southwestern Medical Center, Preventive Cardiology Program

Website: https://utswmed.org/conditions-treatments /preventive-cardiology/

Phone: 214-645-8000

Houston and other locations: Debakey Heart & Vascular Center, Houston Methodist Hospital

Website: https://www.houstonmethodist.org/heart -vascular/prevention/

Phone: 713-332-2539

Plano: Baylor Scott & White The Heart Hospital, Center for Cardiovascular Disease Prevention

Website: https://www.bswhealth.com/the-heart -hospital/locations/plano/center-for-cardiovascular -disease-prevention/

Phone: 469-814-4863

UTAH

Statewide (and Idaho, Wyoming, Montana, and much of Nevada): University of Utah Health

1. Go to the web page: https://healthcare.utah.edu/fad/
2. In the box labeled "I want to see a", choose: Specialist
3. In the box that appears labeled "Specializing in," type and select: preventive cardiology

WISCONSIN

Milwaukee: Froedtert Health and the Medical College of Wisconsin, Preventive Cardiology Program

Website: https://www.froedtert.com/preventive-cardiology-lipid-therapy/doctors

Phone: 414-777-7700

ACKNOWLEDGMENTS

This book was a labor of love, motivated by heart disease in family members that developed long ago, before early diagnosis was available and statin therapy was known to be safe and effective. In a pattern that will be familiar to many readers, heart disease, also known as artery clogging, caused my father's death, my mother's vascular dementia, and my grandmother's debilitating stroke.

I would first like to thank preventive cardiologist Roger Blumenthal for prescribing a statin medication at a dosage that lowered my "bad" LDL cholesterol to a level low enough to stabilize the existing plaque in my arteries and stop further artery clogging, and also my primary care provider who now manages my statin prescription.

To all the medical researchers who chose to publish the journal articles described in this book as free, open access articles: thank you.

My work in journalism has improved my ability to explain complex information in clear language, and so I thank John Fitzgerald Weaver for introducing me to my first editor at PV Magazine USA, and also my editors there over the years: Anne Fischer, Christian Roselund and David Wagman.

Novelist Deborah Wunderman inspired me to update my free online book on this topic to produce the version you are reading. Rick Wunderman engaged in debates on artery clogging and health. Casey Watts shared his experience in publishing a book with Ingram Spark.

My sisters Sheila and Lorraine and my wife Karen served as key early reviewers.

Affordable higher education was the foundation of my writing career, because it made possible my attendance at Yale, Princeton, and George Mason universities. I hope that young people may find increasing opportunities for affordable higher education in the future.

William L. Driscoll

NOTES

For interested readers, note that many of the medical journal articles described in this book are available free online at the links provided below.

Chapter 1: Heart Disease is a Disease of the Arteries

a disease of the arteries: One less common form of heart disease, however, is caused by a problem with the heart valves, not a problem with the arteries.

leading cause of death in the United States: U.S. Centers for Disease Control and Prevention. Leading Causes of Death. Accessed May 10, 2023. https://www.cdc.gov/nchs/fastats/leading-causes-of-death.htm

leading cause of death worldwide: World Health Organization. The top 10 causes of death. Accessed May 10, 2023. https://www.who.int/news-room/fact-sheets/detail/the-top-10-causes-of-death

until they have a heart attack or stroke: Cleveland Clinic. Atherosclerosis. Accessed May 10, 2023. https://my .clevelandclinic.org/health/diseases/16753-atherosclerosis -arterial-disease

failed to prompt statin therapy in 85%: Sánchez-Cabo F, Rossello X, Fuster V, et al. Machine Learning Improves Cardiovascular Risk Definition for Young, Asymptomatic Individuals. *J Am Coll Cardiol.* 2020;76(14):1674-1685. https://doi:10.1016/j.jacc.2020.08.017

"proceed unchecked for decades": Navar AM, Peterson ED. Statin Recommendations for Primary Prevention: More of the Same or Time for a Change? *JAMA.* 2022;328(8):716-718. https://doi:10.1001/jama.2022.12982

image compares a healthy artery: U.S. National Institutes of Health. What is Atherosclerosis? Accessed May 10, 2023. https://www.nhlbi.nih.gov/health/atherosclerosis

if an area of plaque bursts: U.S. National Institutes of Health. What is Atherosclerosis? Accessed May 10, 2023. https://www.nhlbi.nih.gov/health/atherosclerosis

A coronary artery is shown: U.S. Centers for Disease Control and Prevention. Coronary Artery Disease. Accessed May 10, 2023. https://www.cdc.gov/heartdisease /coronary_ad.htm

A carotid artery is shown: U.S. National Institutes of Health. What to Expect When Getting a Stent. Accessed August 16, 2023. https://www.nhlbi.nih.gov/health/stents /during

"poor aging": Makover ME, Shapiro MD, Toth PP. There is urgent need to treat atherosclerotic cardiovascular disease risk earlier, more intensively, and with greater precision: A review of current practice and recommendations for improved effectiveness. *Am J Prev Cardiol.* 2022;12:100371. https://doi:10.1016/j.ajpc.2022.100371

LDL cholesterol causes artery clogging: Libby P. The changing landscape of atherosclerosis. *Nature.* 2021;592(7855):524-533. https://doi:10.1038/s41586-021 -03392-8

identifying this condition: U.S. Preventive Services Task Force. Final Evidence Review—Asymptomatic Carotid Artery Stenosis: Screening. Accessed May 10, 2023. https://www.uspreventiveservicestaskforce.org /uspstf/document/final-evidence-review/carotid-artery -stenosis-screening

Artery clogging can lead to: Makover ME, Shapiro MD, Toth PP. There is urgent need to treat atherosclerotic cardiovascular disease risk earlier, more intensively, and with greater precision: A review of current practice and recommendations for improved effectiveness. *Am J Prev Cardiol.* 2022;12:100371. https://doi:10.1016/j.ajpc.2022.100371

Chapter 2: How Arteries Get Clogged Even With a "Normal" Cholesterol Level

LDL cholesterol causes artery clogging: Ference BA, Ginsberg HN, Graham I, et al. Low-density lipoproteins cause atherosclerotic cardiovascular disease. 1. Evidence from genetic, epidemiologic, and clinical studies. A consensus statement from the European Atherosclerosis Society Consensus Panel. *Eur Heart J.* 2017;38(32):2459-2472. https://doi:10.1093/eurheartj/ehx144

the "strongest modifiable risk factor": López-Melgar B, Fernández-Friera L, Oliva B, et al. Short-Term Progression of Multiterritorial Subclinical Atherosclerosis. *J Am Coll Cardiol.* 2020;75(14):1617-1627. https://doi:10.1016/j.jacc.2020.02.026

if your LDL level is measured in different units: If you live in a part of the world where your LDL level is reported in units of mmol/L, you can convert that measurement to units of mg/dL by multiplying the number of mmol/L by 38.67, according to this source: U.S. National Institutes of Health. Screening and Treatment of Subclinical Hypothyroidism or Hyperthyroidism. Accessed May 10, 2023. https://www.ncbi.nlm.nih.gov/books/NBK83505/

"lower is better": O'Keefe JH Jr, Cordain L, Harris WH, Moe RM, Vogel R. Optimal low-density lipoprotein is 50 to 70 mg/dl: lower is better and physiologically normal. *J Am Coll Cardiol.* 2004;43(11):2142-2146. https://doi:10.1016/j.jacc.2004.03.046

"LDL cholesterol: the lower the better": Martin SS, Blumenthal RS, Miller M. LDL cholesterol: the lower the better [published correction appears in *Med Clin North Am.* 2012 May;96(3):xv-xvi]. *Med Clin North Am.* 2012;96(1):13-26. https://doi:10.1016/j.mcna.2012.01.009

a "3-fold greater reduction": Ference BA, Yoo W, Alesh I, et al. Effect of long-term exposure to lower low-density lipoprotein cholesterol beginning early in life on the risk of coronary heart disease: a Mendelian randomization analysis. *J Am Coll Cardiol.* 2012;60(25):2631-2639. https://doi:10.1016/j.jacc.2012.09.017

"proportional to both the magnitude and the duration": Toth PP. Identification and treatment of those most at risk for premature atherosclerotic cardiovascular disease: We just cannot seem to get it right. *Am J Prev Cardiol.* 2020;2:100040. https://doi:10.1016/j.ajpc.2020.100040

"the earlier elevated LDL cholesterol is lowered, the better": Makover ME, Shapiro MD, Toth PP. There is urgent need to treat atherosclerotic cardiovascular disease risk earlier, more intensively, and with greater precision: A review of current practice and recommendations for improved effectiveness. *Am J Prev Cardiol.* 2022;12:100371. https://doi:10.1016/j.ajpc.2022.100371

LDL levels that can reach as low as 14: Karagiannis AD, Mehta A, Dhindsa DS, et al. How low is safe? The frontier of very low (<30 mg/dL) LDL cholesterol. *Eur Heart J.* 2021;42(22):2154-2169. https://doi:10.1093/eurheartj/ehaa1080

much lower levels of LDL than the level "below 100": Johns Hopkins Medicine. Lipid Panel. Accessed May 10, 2023. https://www.hopkinsmedicine.org/health/treatment-tests-and-therapies/lipid-panel

a standard that dates back to 2008: U.S. Centers for Disease Control and Prevention. National Health and Nutrition Examination Survey 2005-2006 Data Documentation, Codebook, and Frequencies Cholesterol - LDL, Triglyceride & Apoliprotein (ApoB) (TRIGLY_D). Accessed May 10, 2023. https://wwwn.cdc.gov/nchs /nhanes/2005-2006/TRIGLY_D.htm

"should be below 38": Makover ME, Shapiro MD, Toth PP. There is urgent need to treat atherosclerotic cardio-vascular disease risk earlier, more intensively, and with greater precision: A review of current practice and recommendations for improved effectiveness. *Am J Prev Cardiol.* 2022;12:100371. https://doi:10.1016/j.ajpc.2022.100371

the rate of increase in risk "rises more steeply": Grundy SM, Cleeman JI, Merz CN, et al. Implications of recent clinical trials for the National Cholesterol Education Program Adult Treatment Panel III Guidelines. *J Am Coll Cardiol.* 2004;44(3):720-732. https://doi:10.1016/j.jacc .2004.07.001

an LDL level below 55: Mach F, Baigent C, Catapano AL, et al. 2019 ESC/EAS Guidelines for the management of dyslipidaemias: lipid modification to reduce cardiovascular risk [published correction appears in *Eur Heart J.* 2020 Nov 21;41(44):4255]. *Eur Heart J.* 2020;41(1):111-188. https://doi:10.1093/eurheartj/ehz455

"Optimal low-density lipoprotein is 50 to 70": O'Keefe JH Jr, Cordain L, Harris WH, Moe RM, Vogel R. Optimal low-density lipoprotein is 50 to 70 mg/dl: lower is better and physiologically normal. *J Am Coll Cardiol.*

2004;43(11):2142-2146. https://doi:10.1016/j.jacc.2004
.03.046

artery-clogging plaque regressed: In the following article's
central illustration, see the blue line showing a reduction in
"percent atheroma volume," or percentage of artery clog-
ging, at LDL cholesterol levels below 70 md/dL: Tsujita K,
Sugiyama S, Sumida H, et al. Impact of Dual Lipid-
Lowering Strategy With Ezetimibe and Atorvastatin on
Coronary Plaque Regression in Patients With Percutaneous
Coronary Intervention: The Multicenter Randomized
Controlled PRECISE-IVUS Trial. *J Am Coll Cardiol.*
2015;66(5):495-507. https://doi:10.1016/j.jacc.2015.05.065

less than 70: Grundy SM, Stone NJ, Blumenthal RS, et al.
High-Intensity Statins Benefit High-Risk Patients: Why and
How to Do Better. *Mayo Clin Proc.* 2021;96(10):2660-2670.
https://doi:10.1016/j.mayocp.2021.02.032

among those with an LDL level of 70-80: Fernández-Friera
L, Fuster V, López-Melgar B, et al. Normal LDL-Cholesterol
Levels Are Associated With Subclinical Atherosclerosis in
the Absence of Risk Factors [published correction appears
in *J Am Coll Cardiol.* 2018 Feb 6;71(5):588-589]. *J Am
Coll Cardiol.* 2017;70(24):2979-2991. https://doi:10.1016/j
.jacc.2017.10.024

an LDL level below 100 is not protective: Sachdeva A,
Cannon CP, Deedwania PC, et al. Lipid levels in patients
hospitalized with coronary artery disease: an analysis of
136,905 hospitalizations in Get with the Guidelines. *Am
Heart J.* 2009;157(1):111-117.e2. https://doi:10.1016/j
.ahj.2008.08.010

the likelihood of disease or death was 2.97 times higher: Duncan MS, Vasan RS, Xanthakis V. Trajectories of Blood Lipid Concentrations Over the Adult Life Course and Risk of Cardiovascular Disease and All-Cause Mortality: Observations From the Framingham Study Over 35 Years. *J Am Heart Assoc.* 2019 Jun 4;8(11):e011433. https://doi:10.1161/JAHA.118.011433

among those with LDL between 130 and 160: Fernández-Friera L, Fuster V, López-Melgar B, et al. Normal LDL-Cholesterol Levels Are Associated With Subclinical Atherosclerosis in the Absence of Risk Factors [published correction appears in *J Am Coll Cardiol.* 2018 Feb 6;71(5):588-589]. *J Am Coll Cardiol.* 2017;70(24):2979-2991. https://doi:10.1016/j.jacc.2017.10.024

nearly 60% had arterial plaque: Fernández-Friera L, Peñalvo JL, Fernández-Ortiz A, et al. Prevalence, Vascular Distribution, and Multiterritorial Extent of Subclinical Atherosclerosis in a Middle-Aged Cohort: The PESA (Progression of Early Subclinical Atherosclerosis) Study. *Circulation.* 2015;131(24):2104-2113. https://doi:10.1161/CIRCULATIONAHA.114.014310

arterial imaging at an early stage: Nambi V, Bhatt DL. Primary Prevention of Atherosclerosis: Time to Take a Selfie? *J Am Coll Cardiol.* 2017;70(24):2992-2994. https://doi:10.1016/j.jacc.2017.10.068

for every 30 mg/dL increase in the LDL level: Grundy SM, Cleeman JI, Merz CN, et al. Implications of recent clinical trials for the National Cholesterol Education

Program Adult Treatment Panel III Guidelines. *J Am Coll Cardiol*. 2004;44(3):720-732. https://doi:10.1016/j.jacc.2004.07.001

LDL of 190 or higher: Grundy S, Stone N, Bailey A, et al. 2018 AHA/ACC/AACVPR/AAPA/ABC/ACPM/ADA/AGS/APhA/ASPC/NLA/PCNA Guideline on the Management of Blood Cholesterol: Executive Summary. *J Am Coll Cardiol*. 2019 Jun; 73(24):3168–3209. https://doi.org/10.1016/j.jacc.2018.11.002

the following table may be helpful: The table is based on: Mayo Clinic. Cholesterol Test. Accessed August 21, 2023. https://www.mayoclinic.org/tests-procedures/cholesterol-test/about/pac-20384601

Chapter 3: Limiting Artery Clogging at an Early Stage Can Protect Your Health

A blood clot in an artery: U.S. National Institutes of Health. What is Atherosclerosis? Accessed May 10, 2023. https://www.nhlbi.nih.gov/health/atherosclerosis

artery clogging can also lead to four other diseases: U.S. National Institutes of Health. What is Atherosclerosis? Accessed May 10, 2023. https://www.nhlbi.nih.gov/health/atherosclerosis

peripheral artery disease: U.S. National Institutes of Health. Peripheral Artery Disease: Living With. Accessed May 10, 2023. https://www.nhlbi.nih.gov/health/peripheral-artery-disease/living-with

renal artery "stenosis": U.S. National Institutes of Health. Renal Artery Stenosis. Accessed May 10, 2023. https://www.niddk.nih.gov/health-information/kidney-disease/renal-artery-stenosis

mesenteric artery ischemia: U.S. National Institutes of Health. Mesenteric artery ischemia. Accessed May 10, 2023. https://medlineplus.gov/ency/article/001156.htm

impaired sexual response and "poor aging": Makover ME, Shapiro MD, Toth PP. There is urgent need to treat atherosclerotic cardiovascular disease risk earlier, more intensively, and with greater precision: A review of current practice and recommendations for improved effectiveness. *Am J Prev Cardiol.* 2022;12:100371. https://doi:10.1016/j.ajpc.2022.100371

can slow down the brain: Cortes-Canteli M, Gispert JD, Salvadó G, et al. Subclinical Atherosclerosis and Brain Metabolism in Middle-Aged Individuals: The PESA Study. *J Am Coll Cardiol.* 2021;77(7):888-898. https://doi:10.1016/j.jacc.2020.12.027

Chapter 4: Should You Get Tested for Artery Clogging?

Five cardiologists (heart doctors) have proposed: Ahmadi A, Argulian E, Leipsic J, Newby DE, Narula J. From Subclinical Atherosclerosis to Plaque Progression and Acute Coronary Events: JACC State-of-the-Art Review. *J Am Coll Cardiol.* 2019;74(12):1608-1617. https://doi:10.1016/j.jacc.2019.08.012

scoring is based on several factors: American College of Cardiology. ASCVD Risk Estimator Plus. Accessed May 10, 2023. https://tools.acc.org/ascvd-risk-estimator-plus/#! /calculate/estimate/

risk scoring failed to trigger preventive treatment: Sánchez-Cabo F, Rossello X, Fuster V, et al. Machine Learning Improves Cardiovascular Risk Definition for Young, Asymptomatic Individuals. *J Am Coll Cardiol.* 2020;76(14):1674-1685. https://doi:10.1016/j.jacc.2020.08.017

"nearly 60%" of those classified as having low risk: Fernández-Friera L, Peñalvo JL, Fernández-Ortiz A, et al. Prevalence, Vascular Distribution, and Multiterritorial Extent of Subclinical Atherosclerosis in a Middle-Aged Cohort: The PESA (Progression of Early Subclinical Atherosclerosis) Study. *Circulation.* 2015;131(24):2104-2113. https://doi:10.1161/CIRCULATIONAHA.114.014310

"allows atherosclerosis to proceed unchecked for decades": Navar AM, Peterson ED. Statin Recommendations for Primary Prevention: More of the Same or Time for a Change? *JAMA.* 2022;328(8):716-718. https:// doi:10.1001/jama.2022.12982

actually took a statin medication: Patel N, Bhargava A, Kalra R, et al. Trends in Lipid, Lipoproteins, and Statin Use Among U.S. Adults: Impact of 2013 Cholesterol Guidelines. *J Am Coll Cardiol.* 2019;74(20):2525-2528. https://doi:10.1016/j.jacc.2019.09.026

proposed that primary care providers test people: Ahmadi A, Argulian E, Leipsic J, Newby DE, Narula J.

From Subclinical Atherosclerosis to Plaque Progression and Acute Coronary Events: JACC State-of-the-Art Review. *J Am Coll Cardiol.* 2019;74(12):1608-1617. https://doi:10.1016/j.jacc.2019.08.012

screening "at the earliest age possible": Makover ME, Shapiro MD, Toth PP. There is urgent need to treat atherosclerotic cardiovascular disease risk earlier, more intensively, and with greater precision: A review of current practice and recommendations for improved effectiveness. *Am J Prev Cardiol.* 2022;12:100371. https://doi:10.1016/j.ajpc.2022.100371

an "independent, volunteer panel": U.S. Preventive Services Task Force. Home page. Accessed May 21, 2023. https://www.uspreventiveservicestaskforce.org/uspstf/

"may potentially lead to changes in medical management": U.S. Preventive Services Task Force. Final Evidence Review—Asymptomatic Carotid Artery Stenosis: Screening. Accessed May 10, 2023. https://www.uspreventiveservicestaskforce.org/uspstf/document/final-evidence-review/carotid-artery-stenosis-screening

only surgical treatment of advanced artery clogging: The task force recommended against carotid artery screening because, the final evidence review said, preventing deaths through changes in medical management, such as statin therapy, was "outside the scope" of its review.

"may provide incremental information": Sengupta PP, Andrikopoulou E, Choi AD, et al. Cardiovascular Point of Care Ultrasound: Current Value and Vision for Future

Use. American College of Cardiology. Accessed May 12, 2023. https://ww.acc.org/About-ACC/Innovation/POCUS

for those with diabetes aged 40-75: American College of Cardiology. Key Points From the 2019 ACC/AHA Guidelines on the Primary Prevention of Cardiovascular Disease. Accessed May 10, 2023. https://www.acc.org /latest-in-cardiology/articles/2019/04/29/07/42/key -points-from-the-2019-acc-aha-guidelines-on-the-primary -prevention-of-cvd

among otherwise healthy people with LDL above 130: Fernández-Friera L, Fuster V, López-Melgar B, et al. Normal LDL-Cholesterol Levels Are Associated With Subclinical Atherosclerosis in the Absence of Risk Factors [published correction appears in *J Am Coll Cardiol.* 2018 Feb 6;71(5):588-589]. *J Am Coll Cardiol.* 2017;70(24):2979-2991. https://doi:10.1016/j.jacc.2017.10.024

Even a mild form of high blood pressure: Nam KW, Kwon HM, Jeong HY, Park JH, Kwon H, Jeong SM. Intracranial Atherosclerosis and Stage 1 Hypertension Defined by the 2017 ACC/AHA Guideline. *Am J Hypertens.* 2020;33(1):92-98. https://doi:10.1093/ajh/hpz138

systolic blood pressure of 120-129: Whelton SP, McEvoy JW, Shaw L, et al. Association of Normal Systolic Blood Pressure Level With Cardiovascular Disease in the Absence of Risk Factors. *JAMA Cardiol.* 2020;5(9):1011-1018. https://doi:10.1001/jamacardio.2020.1731

a doctor "may recommend": Mayo Clinic. Carotid ultrasound. Accessed May 10, 2023. https://www.mayoclinic

.org/tests-procedures/carotid-ultrasound/about/pac
-20393399

"if you have high blood pressure": Cleveland Clinic. Carotid Ultrasound. Accessed May 10, 2023. https://my .clevelandclinic.org/health/diagnostics/22916-carotid -ultrasound

The directions are available: Centers for Disease Control and Prevention. Measuring Your Blood Pressure. Accessed August 5, 2023. https://www.cdc.gov/bloodpressure /measure.htm

Black Americans had a higher prevalence of strokes: Thorpe RJ Jr, Fesahazion RG, Parker L, et al. Accelerated Health Declines among African Americans in the USA. *J Urban Health*. 2016;93(5):808-819. https://doi:10.1007 /s11524-016-0075-4

those who have one or more of six risk factors: Toth PP. Identification and treatment of those most at risk for pre-mature atherosclerotic cardiovascular disease: We just cannot seem to get it right. *Am J Prev Cardiol*. 2020;2:100040. https://doi:10.1016/j.ajpc.2020.100040

Other "risk enhancers": American College of Cardiol-ogy. Key Points From the 2019 ACC/ AHA Guidelines on the Primary Prevention of Cardiovascular Disease. Accessed May 10, 2023. https://www.acc.org/latest-in -cardiology/articles/2019/04/29/07/42/key-points-from -the-2019-acc-aha-guidelines-on-the-primary-prevention -of-cvd

those with a "low socioeconomic status": Woolsey AB, Arsang-Jang S, Spence JD, Hackam DG, Azarpazhooh MR. The impact of socioeconomic status on the burden of atherosclerosis, and the effect of intensive preventive therapy on its progression: A retrospective cohort study. *Atherosclerosis*. 2022;358:29-33. https://doi:10.1016/j.atherosclerosis.2022.08.013

People with sleep apnea: Walia HK, Khosla AA, Saxena A, et al. Atherosclerotic plaque in individuals without known cardiovascular disease but with established obstructive sleep apnea and at high risk of obstructive sleep apnea. *Am J Prev Cardiol*. 2023;14:100497. https://doi.org/10.1016/j.ajpc.2023.100497

"Erectile dysfunction is a marker": Miner M, Nehra A, Jackson G, et al. All men with vasculogenic erectile dysfunction require a cardiovascular workup. *Am J Med*. 2014;127(3):174-182. https://doi:10.1016/j.amjmed.2013.10.013

cumulative prior exposure to LDL cholesterol: Domanski MJ, Tian X, Wu CO, et al. Time Course of LDL Cholesterol Exposure and Cardiovascular Disease Event Risk. *J Am Coll Cardiol*. 2020;76(13):1507-1516. https://doi:10.1016/j.jacc.2020.07.059

5,000 mg-years of LDL "seems to be the tipping point": American College of Cardiology. Latest in Cardiology. Dyslipidemia Over a Lifetime: The Case for Early Intervention on LDL Cholesterol. Accessed August 5, 2023 https://www.acc.org/latest-in-cardiology/articles/2018/10/11/08/41/dyslipidemia-over-a-lifetime

Artery clogging progressed "significantly": López-Melgar B, Fernández-Friera L, Oliva B, et al. Short-Term Progression of Multiterritorial Subclinical Atherosclerosis. *J Am Coll Cardiol.* 2020;75(14):1617-1627. https://doi:10.1016/j.jacc.2020.02.026

screening "is appropriate": Life Line Screening. Carotid Artery Disease Screening. Accessed May 10, 2023. https://www.lifelinescreening.com/screening-services/carotid-artery-disease-screening

free artery screenings: Dare to CARE. Accessed December 16, 2023. https://hearthealthfoundation.org/dare-to-care/

over 90% were considered "positive" for artery clogging: Wong ND, Lopez VA, Allison M, et al. Abdominal aortic calcium and multi-site atherosclerosis: the Multiethnic Study of Atherosclerosis. *Atherosclerosis.* 2011;214(2):436-441. https://doi:10.1016/j.atherosclerosis.2010.09.011

free artery screenings for anyone over 60: Dare to CARE. Accessed December 16, 2023. https://hearthealthfoundation.org/dare-to-care/

screening "at the earliest age possible": Makover ME, Shapiro MD, Toth PP. There is urgent need to treat atherosclerotic cardiovascular disease risk earlier, more intensively, and with greater precision: A review of current practice and recommendations for improved effectiveness. *Am J Prev Cardiol.* 2022;12:100371. https://doi.org/10.1016/j.ajpc.2022.100371

a "significantly increased" likelihood: Gupta A, Lau E, Varshney R, et al. The identification of calcified coronary plaque is associated with initiation and continuation of pharmacological and lifestyle preventive therapies: A systematic review and meta-analysis. JACC Cardiovasc Imaging. 2017;10(8):833–842. https://doi.org/10.1016/j .jcmg.2017.01.030

Chapter 5: How to Get Tested for Artery Clogging

without an order from your doctor: Author's personal communication with a Life Line Screening representative. May 10, 2023.

And: Dare to CARE. Accessed December 16, 2023. https:// hearthealthfoundation.org/dare-to-care/

And: Atrium Health Navicent. Why AngioScreen? Accessed August 1, 2023. https://navicenthealth.org/service-center /heart-and-vascular-care/why-angioscreen

based largely on the speed of blood flow: Life Line Screening. Carotid artery disease screening (video). Accessed May 10, 2023. https://www.lifelinescreening .com/screening-services/carotid-artery-disease-screening

And: Dare to C.A.R.E. Carotid artery duplex. Accessed May 10, 2023. https://www.daretocare.us/about-the -program/c-a-r-e-screenings/carotid-artery-duplex/

And: Atrium Health Navicent. Accessed July 24, 2023. https://navicent-health.org/js/tinymce/plugins/filemanager /files/the-georgia-heart-center/SAMPLE_REPORT.pdf

about 40 other U.S. health care systems: These health care systems were identified by the author through a Google search on the phrase "screening of the arteries" on July 21, 2023.

or has mild, moderate or severe clogging: Life Line Screening. Understanding Your Health Screening Results. Accessed August 3, 2023. https://www.lifelinescreening .com/wp-content/uploads/2021/10/13_About-your-results _Mod-1_Results.pdf

carotid artery ultrasound screening test for $85: Author's personal communication with a Life Line Screening representative, April 26, 2023.

offers free carotid artery ultrasound screening: Heart Health Foundation. Accessed December 16, 2023. https:// hearthealthfoundation.org/

Dare to CARE scheduling: Locations. Accessed December 16, 2023. https://hearthealthfoundation.org/locations/

offers screening in the Midwest: Author's personal communication with a Health Gauge Screenings participant, September 29, 2023.

incorporates the use of a contrast dye: Atrium Health Navicent. Atrium Health Navicent Offers AngioScreening For Early Heart Disease Detection. Accessed August 3, 2023. https://navicenthealth.org/community/single_news /atrium-health-navicent-offers-angioscreening-for-early -heart-disease-detection

shows the extent of carotid artery blockage: Atrium Health Navicent. Sample Report. Accessed July 24, 2023. https://navicenthealth.org/js/tinymce/plugins /filemanager/files/the-georgia-heart-center/SAMPLE _REPORT.pdf

Atrium Health Navicent scheduling: Atrium Health Navicent. Atrium Health Navicent Heart & Vascular Care. Accessed July 31, 2023. https://navicenthealth.org /service-center/heart-and-vascular-care/schedule

have not publicly disclosed: These health care systems, identified by the author through a Google search on the phrase "screening of the arteries" on July 21, 2023, did not disclose on their screening program web page whether they report early-stage artery clogging to screening participants.

American College of Cardiology workbook: Sengupta PP, Andrikopoulou E, Choi AD, et al. Cardiovascular Point of Care Ultrasound: Current Value and Vision for Future Use. Accessed May 12, 2023. https://www.acc.org /About-ACC/Innovation/POCUS

handheld ultrasound devices: American College of Emergency Physicians. Policy Statement: Appropriate Use Criteria for Handheld/Pocket Ultrasound Devices. Accessed May 10, 2023. https://www.acep.org/globalassets /new-pdfs/policy-statements/appropriate-use-criteria-for -handheld-pocket-ultrasound-devices.pdf

At least eight different brands: Malik AN, Rowland J, Haber BD, et al. The Use of Handheld Ultrasound Devices in Emergency Medicine. *Curr Emerg Hosp Med Rep*. 2021;9(3):73-81. https://doi:10.1007/s40138-021-00229-6

a free follow-up screening in five years: Dare to CARE Eligibility. Accessed May 10, 2023. https://www.daretocare .us/about-the-program/eligibility/

three other tests: Ahmadi A, Argulian E, Leipsic J, Newby DE, Narula J. From Subclinical Atherosclerosis to Plaque Progression and Acute Coronary Events: JACC State-of-the-Art Review. *J Am Coll Cardiol*. 2019;74(12):1608-1617. https://doi:10.1016/j.jacc.2019.08.012

superior to a CAC test: In the following open-access article, see the bottom two charts of figure 1: Rossello X, Raposeiras-Roubin S, Oliva B, et al. Glycated Hemoglobin and Subclinical Atherosclerosis in People Without Diabetes. *J Am Coll Cardiol*. 2021;77(22):2777-2791. https://doi:10.1016/j.jacc.2021.03.335

"calcification" of an artery: Razavi AC, Mehta A, Sperling LS. Statin therapy for the primary prevention of cardiovascular disease: Pros. *Atherosclerosis*. 2022;356:41-45. https:// doi:10.1016/j.atherosclerosis.2022.07.004

Chapter 6: If You Have Artery Clogging: Healthy Choices

The American Heart Association promotes: American Heart Association. Life's Essential 8™. Accessed May 10, 2023. https://www.heart.org/en/healthy-living/healthy -lifestyle/lifes-essential-8

The "optimal" diet: Belardo D, Michos ED, Blankstein R, et al. Practical, Evidence-Based Approaches to Nutritional Modifications to Reduce Atherosclerotic Cardiovascular Disease: An American Society For Preventive Cardiology Clinical Practice Statement. *Am J Prev Cardiol.* 2022; 10:100323. https://doi:10.1016/j.ajpc.2022.100323

ultra-processed foods: Martínez Steele E, Baraldi LG, Louzada ML, Moubarac JC, Mozaffarian D, Monteiro CA. Ultra-processed foods and added sugars in the US diet: evidence from a nationally representative cross-sectional study. *BMJ Open.* 2016;6(3):e009892. https://doi:10.1136 /bmjop-en-2015-009892

vegans need vitamin B-12: Melina V, Craig W, Levin S. Position of the Academy of Nutrition and Dietetics: Vegetarian Diets. *J Acad Nutr Diet.* 2016;116(12):1970-1980. https://doi:10.1016/j.jand.2016.09.025

The American Heart Association favors: Gardner CD, Vadiveloo MK, Petersen KS, et al. Popular Dietary Patterns: Alignment With American Heart Association 2021 Dietary Guidance: A Scientific Statement From the American Heart Association [published online ahead of print, 2023 Apr 27]. *Circulation.* 2023;10.1161/CIR.0000000000001146. https:// doi:10.1161/CIR.0000000000001146

Chapter 7: If You Have Artery Clogging: Statin Therapy

Statin drugs stabilize vulnerable plaques: Ahmadi A, Argulian E, Leipsic J, Newby DE, Narula J. From

Subclinical Atherosclerosis to Plaque Progression and Acute Coronary Events: JACC State-of-the-Art Review. *J Am Coll Cardiol.* 2019;74(12):1608–1617. https://doi .org/10.1016/j.jacc.2019.08.012

lipid-lowering therapy can "halt" the progression of plaque: Ahmadi A, Argulian E, Leipsic J, Newby DE, Narula J. From subclinical atherosclerosis to plaque progression and acute coronary events: JACC state-of-the-art review. *J Am Coll Cardiol.* 2019;74(12):1608–1617. https:// doi.org/10.1016/j.jacc.2019.08.012

artery-clogging plaque regressed: In the following article's central illustration, see the blue line showing a reduction in "percent atheroma volume," or percentage of artery clogging, at LDL cholesterol levels below 70 md/dL: Tsujita K, Sugiyama S, Sumida H, et al. Impact of dual lipid-lowering strategy with ezetimibe and atorvastatin on coronary plaque regression in patients with percutaneous coronary intervention: The multicenter randomized controlled PRECISE-IVUS trial. *J Am Coll Cardiol.* 2015;66(5):495–507. https://doi.org/10.1016/j.jacc.2015.05.065

"significant reductions" in a plaque component: Brinjikji W, Lehman VT, Kallmes DF, et al. The effects of statin therapy on carotid plaque composition and volume: A systematic review and meta-analysis. *J Neuroradiol.* 2017;44(4):234-240. https://doi.org/10.1016/j .neurad.2016.12.004

"high-intensity" or "moderate-intensity": Mach F, Baigent C, Catapano AL, et al. 2019 ESC/EAS guidelines for the management of dyslipidaemias: Lipid modification to reduce cardiovascular risk: The Task Force for the Management of Dyslipidaemias of the European Society of Cardiology (ESC) and European Atherosclerosis Society (EAS). *Eur Heart J.* 2020;41(1):111–1881. https://doi .org/10.1093/eurheartj/ehz455

Chapter 8: How Safe Are Statins?

"usually well tolerated and safe": Grundy S, Stone N, Bailey A, et al. 2018 AHA/ACC/AACVPR/AAPA/ABC/ ACPM/ADA/AGS/APhA/ASPC/NLA/PCNA guideline on the management of blood cholesterol: Executive summary. *J Am Coll Cardiol.* 2019 Jun;73(24):3168–3209. https://doi .org/10.1016/j.jacc.2018.11.002

Rhabdomyolysis: U.S. Centers for Disease Control and Prevention. Rhabdomyolysis. Accessed May 10, 2023. https://www.cdc.gov/niosh/topics/rhabdo/default.html

The Mayo Clinic advises: Mayo Clinic. Rhabdomyolysis from statins: What's the risk? Accessed May 10, 2023. https:// www.mayoclinic.org/diseases-conditions/high-blood -cholesterol/expert-answers/rhabdomyolysis/faq-20057817

table 11 provides more detail on side effects: AHA/ACC/ AACVPR/AAPA/ABC/ACPM/ADA/AGS/APhA/ASPC/ NLA/PCNA guideline on the management of blood cho- lesterol: Executive summary. Table 11. *J Am Coll Cardiol.* 2019 Jun;73(24):3168–3209. https://www.sciencedirect.com /science/article/pii/S0735109718390338?via%-3Dihub#tbl11

Adverse effects of statin therapy are rare: Visseren FLJ, Mach F, Smulders YM, et al. 2021 ESC guidelines

on cardiovascular disease prevention in clinical practice [published correction appears in Eur Heart J. 2022
Nov 7;43(42):4468]. *Eur Heart J.* 2021;42(34):3227–3337.
https://doi.org/10.1093/eurheartj/ehab484

the primary symptom of myopathy: Penn Medicine.
Myopathies. Accessed May 10, 2023. https://www.penn
medicine.org/for-patients-and-visitors/patient-information
/conditions-treated-a-to-z/myopathies

Chapter 9: When to Seek Out
a Preventive Cardiologist

No references were used for this chapter.

INDEX